Bioidentical Hormone Replacement Therapy

The Naturally Balanced Solution to Hormone Replacement

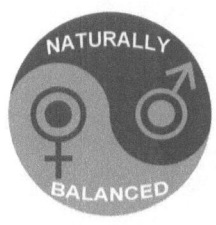

Rudy Dragone, R.PH.

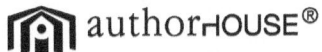
authorHOUSE®

AuthorHouse™ LLC
1663 Liberty Drive
Bloomington, IN 47403
www.authorhouse.com
Phone: 1-800-839-8640

Published by AuthorHouse 02/13/2014

ISBN: 978-1-4389-7618-1 (sc)
ISBN: 978-1-4389-7619-8 (e)

Any people depicted in stock imagery provided by Thinkstock are models, and such images are being used for illustrative purposes only. Certain stock imagery © Thinkstock.

This book is printed on acid-free paper.

Because of the dynamic nature of the Internet, any web addresses or links contained in this book may have changed since publication and may no longer be valid. The views expressed in this work are solely those of the author and do not necessarily reflect the views of the publisher, and the publisher hereby disclaims any responsibility for them.

Table of Contents

Dedicated to God,
with whom all things
are possible.

Educate, Evaluate and Expand

Everywhere you turn these days you hear and see more and more news and advertising about Hormone Replacement Therapies (HRTs). From large pharmaceuticals marketing the latest synthetic low testosterone replacement roll-on to celebrities extolling the virtues of Bioidentical Hormone Replacement Therapy, (BHRT) as a virtual fountain of youth.

The truth is there are a lot of mistruths about the role bioidentical hormones can have in the cure of several severe symptoms; the overall wellbeing of your patients and safety concerns about their use.

This book is to serve as a guide to understanding the role hormones have in assessing symptoms that may be aggravated by hormonal imbalances or deficiencies. The last half of this book contains a clinical reference guide to help healthcare practitioners check for hormonal imbalances and recommend dosing of bioidentical hormones in the treatment of their patients.

The goals of this book are to:
1. Educate healthcare professionals about the role of hormones in the wellness of their patients.
2. Educate the public of the significant role hormonal imbalances can play in their overall wellness.
3. Provide the necessary tools to determine if bioidentical hormone replacement therapies are appropriate for your patients.
4. Help expand healthcare practices through referrals by happy, healthy patients and bioidentical hormone replacement therapies that improve patient lives while making sound business sense to your practice.

The majority of the content in this book is taken directly from lectures and talks that compounding pharmacist and bioidentical hormone replacement therapy expert, Rudy Dragone has given to doctors, fire departments, police departments and thousands of others across the United States and around the globe.

Rudy had worked for years with Dr. William R. Lee, an internationally acknowledged pioneer in the study and use of hormone replacement therapy for women. Together, they were instrumental in the educating thousands of healthcare professionals about the role of hormones and the use of BHRT in healthcare. The fire department in Phoenix Arizona was so impressed; they approved the use and coverage of BHRT in the healthcare of their employees.

The roll that bioidentical hormone replacement therapy has in overall wellbeing for millions of people is simply remarkable.

Background Experience

In life, we have to take care of ourselves. Sometimes in helping others, we neglect what's important in our own lives. If you've ever flown, you've heard the flight attendant spiel about putting on your own oxygen mask first before helping others. Well, this is what I'm trying to help you to do in this book. I want you to help yourself be as healthy and complete as you can be and I'm going to show you some ways to work towards this so that you can help everybody else in your family feel and live a lot better too.

My name is Rudy Dragone and I am a compounding pharmacist. I'll give you a little background of who I am so that when listen to me you start saying to yourself, "Do I want to believe this guy or not?" You will at least have some background knowledge of who I am.

I am a pharmacist. That's all I ever wanted to be. When I was nine years old; my parents put me in a pharmacy in the Bronx. They said this is where we want you to be. We want you off the streets, away from the gangs and everything else that goes with it. So by the time I was 17 I was enrolled in pharmacy school and by the time I was 21, I was the youngest pharmacist in New York City.

When I was at the pharmacy in New York, I used to look up to this one person that had 5 pharmacies in the same neighborhood. I said to myself, "If I ever could have 5 stores, I would be somebody." By 1988, I had ten stores. Then, I sold everything I owned in New York and came to Arizona to retire.

But I couldn't retire from the desire to keep helping people so I bought another pharmacy in Carefree, Arizona just to keep my hands in it and make a positive impact in the wellbeing of my fellow man. It was during this time I met a true pioneer in development of hormone replacement therapies who had been working in the hormone replacement field for about 10 years, Dr. William Lee. Dr. Lee also had a significant role in developing a health program for the Phoenix Fire Department.

Hormones

Natural hormones, it's almost a miracle so few people know so little about them. Why don't more people know more about them? It cannot be patented. Not like Viagra or anything you see on television these days. Natural hormones cannot be patented because they occur naturally in nature. They were found in the 1930s. Because they cannot be patented none of the drug companies make them because they can't make the big money off of them. In fact, they actually take the same identical hormones that should be in your body and change them so they can patent them, package it and sell it.

We are totally against that. We are saying, "This is what God gave you, this is what Mother Nature gave you, and we want to give you the identical hormone that is in your body to begin with to cure your symptoms."

It just makes plain sense doesn't it? Replace the natural hormones that you lose through the years with the same bioidentical hormones that are already found in your body.

Suzanne Sommers has been advocating the use of bioidentical hormones for some time now. More recently Oprah Winfrey and Dr. Oz have been touting the virtues of bioidentical hormones and keeping hormonal balance as a key to good health and wellbeing. So we have a good strong people as our advocate.

Today, I still compound bioidentical hormones specifically tailored to the unique hormonal needs of each and every patient for doctors around the country and internationally. I get calls all day long from doctors and healthcare provider about solutions to vexing medical problems that are easily solved through the proper use of BHRTs.

The words "proper use of BHRTs" is critical here because hormone replacement therapy, whether it is through synthetics or bioidentical hormone replace is not a one size fits all approach. Unfortunately for you and your patients, major pharmaceutical companies cannot tailor their dosing specifically to your patients' needs. Additionally, any hormone replacement therapy should include frequent and thorough testing and adjustments until each patient is in perfect hormonal balance. A "one pill fits all" approach with synthetics is simply not possible. However, working with a compounding pharmacist like myself, you can dial in the specific needs of each and every patient presenting with symptoms aggravated by hormonal imbalances or deficiencies.

When you get to understand everything that I'm going to be talking to you about, I know you will see the benefits that bioidentical hormone replacement can have in your practice and with the overall quality of your patients' lives. We're going to talk about things that are very sensitive; we're going to talk about things that are not so sensitive. By the time we finish, I will guarantee, you will not look to the person to the right or to left of you in the same manner as when you started. I guarantee, that when you go home, you will look at your spouses, you will look at your parents, you will look at everybody you associate yourself with in a different light and hopefully, if I've done my job correctly, you will be able to help those people.

For me it's not about making money. It's about helping people. I pray, I say a little prayer before every lecture because I really believe in this stuff. This stuff has changed my life. And by the time I'm finished with you, you'll see why I'm such an advocate of using bioidentical hormones to help people's lives.

Beginning with the basics; what are hormones? Hormones are the architects that read the DNA and constantly rebuild the body.

Hormones are chemicals that are secreted in the body by glands. There are over 100 of them. They are secreted in the body by glands that have their effect on target tissue.

Let's make believe that we are a one cell organism right now. On the outside of the cell there are all of these locks. A hormone is a key. The hormone key goes in, fits into a particular lock and then turns the lock. When that lock is turned it sends a message to the DNA at the very heart of the cell and it will actually change the DNA. It can alter the DNA and start metabolic processes.

When we were conceived, originally, we were one cell. Then due to a hormonal interaction, that 1 cell becomes 2 cells, 2 cells become 4 cells and eventually those cells began to differentiate. Soon there are bone cells and eye cells and hair cells and everything else that makes us up. There is a pattern by which these things come out. And the way that comes out is because of our hormones.

Hormones can actually take an embryo that is inherently female and turn it to a male. Guys, I hate to tell you this; but at one time we were all female then at a certain point you became man.

Hormones unlocked the secret of the XY chromosomes during the fetal period of development.

Chromosomes are affected by hormones and if you think the synthetics hormones don't affect your chromosomes, you're very, very mistaken. Given a choice between synthetic and natural hormones, bioidentical natural hormones are the way to go.

Premarin Conversion

A woman came in to my pharmacy and said she had been on Premarin 0.625 mg for 10 years and before that she tried everything to relive her perimenopausal symptoms. Even though she still suffered from hot flashes, this is what she thought worked for her.

Then one day her daughter came to one of our seminars about BHRTs and now here is skeptical mom giving us a shot. "I can't believe that you guys can make anything better but my daughter says I should try so here I am" she explained.

I quickly told her about the risks of taking Premarin for so long and how much better natural hormone replacement will work for her. She told me that when she first started she was put on the 0.625 mg and went from 30-50 hot flashes a day to 5 a day. Then the doctor put her on the .9 mg and she began to have breast tenderness and break through bleeding.

She said, "If my choices are 5 hot flashes a day or break through bleeding and sore breasts, I'll take the 5 hot flashes a day!" and there she remained for 10 years with 5 hot flashes a day.

So we got her on a bioidentical hormone replacement therapy and awhile later she came in and said after using the treatment for 1 month that, "Your stuff is not as good as the Premarin. I went from 5 to 10 hot flashes a day!"

I said okay let me talk to the doctor about raising your Estrogen. We error on the side of safety and the Estrogen was raised.

The following month she came in and said, "Your stuff is just as good as Premarin. I have about 5 hot flashes a day."

Again, I said wait a minute and we again raised it just a little bit. The month passed and she came in again and I asked her how she was doing and she remarked, "I cannot believe it. ZERO hot flashes!" For 10 years she dealt with 5 hot flashes a day and now they were gone.

All those years of suffering through hot flashes because her synthetic Premarin hormone treatment regime wasn't tailored to her specifics needs could have been alleviated by a regiment of bioidentical hormones created to bring her body into a natural balance.

One Size Does Not Fit All

A perfect example of a "one size fits all" approach to the management of hormonal imbalances happens when we look at the range of what falls into "normal" when patients present with problems caused by their thyroid levels.

Let's say the range for the average person's thyroid falls between a 1 to a 10. If a patient who is at a 9 for most of his or her life drops down to a 2, their thyroid is still considered to be normal. For that patient, the quality of their life after this shift in what is considered normal for everyone else is anything but normal to them. They feel like crap.

One of the problems with conventional medicine today is that our testing parameters are off. Let me explain. If you go to a doctor, the doctor will say, your thyroid levels should be between

1 and 10. If you fall in the 2, he's going to tell you your thyroid is okay. He's going to pat you on the head and send you home. But you should say, "Wait a minute, I remember when I was younger, I could eat whatever I wanted, and I was always warm and never gained a pound. Now all of a sudden I just look down the Twinkie aisle and POOF my thighs start to pop out or my belly starts to pop out. Why is that happening? And I'm always cold, my hands are cold, my feet are cold, everything is bothering me, why am I so cold? My nails are brittle, my hair is breaking. I wasn't like that. Then I go to the doctor and the doctor tells me I'm okay. How can that be?"

Here is the first problem. Where did this range of what is consider to be a normal thyroid level come from? Well, every lab has different levels. The reason why every lab has different levels is because they take a look at the people that come in for a thyroid test and they make an average of where they should be or what is "normal".

Well, first things first, the people that are going to be tested for thyroid are being sent to the lab because they have signs of thyroid deficiency or are being tested because the symptoms they present are symptomatic of a hormone imbalance or a deficiency. So right off the bat, if you take a look at all the people who had thyroid symptoms, of course the levels are going to be lower then what should be in your body.

Then there's a second problem. Let's say you're 14, 15, 19, 21 years of age and you're running at a 9 in the thyroid range. All your life you never get tested. Why? Because you didn't have a thyroid problem all those years. You were warm, your body was consuming the food and everything felt great! Right?

Now you go to the doctor and you're a 2 on the thyroid range table. He's going to say you fell into the normal range. The truth of the matter is that a level of 2 is not normal for your body. Your body was used to running at a 9, now it's a 2. Therefore, you can't run your body the way you used to. You can use this example I'm giving here about thyroid and do it to all the hormones.

These hormonal imbalances reach well beyond the effect they have on an individual and can adversely affect those around them.

I love this example of a broken screen door. A woman, her husband and three children walked into the pharmacy and explained that she had been to many doctors and that no one had been able to help her. She had a full hysterectomy and at 28 and was in full blown menopause.

I have to add that she looked exhausted and so did the husband. The children looked unkempt. We started her on the program and helped her in achieving hormonal balance.

Several months passed and one day the whole family was in picking up her prescription. The husband and wife looked happy. Children were clean, orderly and well behaved. They saw me working in the back and asked to talk to me. After expressing their gratitude for helping her, he shared this story with me.

He said their life before the natural hormones was on the rocks. He said he had a screen door on the outside of their home and everyday he would kick it open and slam it shut so it was in terrible shape; holes in the screen and the door hanging loosely by the hinges.

But, that was before natural hormones. Once his wife got on the hormones, she started to feel better, she started to do more housework and look after the children. So he started to do the same. Soon this working together led to sex and not just sex but good loving sex. Soon he fixed the screen door. He tells me he did not realize it then but that broken down door stood there as a testament to how bad their marriage was. Now the new door is a sign of how good their marriage is.

Quality of Life

What happens to the quality of our life as we age? We start with a certain quality of life that changes through the years.

When we're younger we maintain a decent quality. Then all of a sudden in our 30s and 40s we start to drop down. This quality can be maintained a little further out depending on if you do more exercise or if you do less exercise, if you're taking the right vitamins, or eating correctly, or drinking alcohol, or drinking coffee, all of these things have a factor. They can push this line this way or that way.

Do the right things, you can push it up this way. Do the bad things, you're pushing it down this way. That's all that is. But what is happening is the average person will start to slope down and at a certain point they just bounce along the bottom and they die.

If you see the older people, they are always complaining I have this hurting me, that hurting me, I'm not happy. Why doesn't the Lord take me and it'll make it easier on me? If you ever heard that, you probably will. This is what people do. I'm fighting that. I'm saying this is not the way it should be.

Take a look at a fruit fly. A fruit fly has a great quality of life. It only lives 28 days but it will go full quality of life for 28 days and then it'll die.

What we're about is not that we found the fountain of youth. What we think we did is found the fountain of health. When we look at patients now, instead of looking at them as a fibromyalgia patient, or a systemic lupus erythematous patient, we look at them as a patient that may have a hormone imbalance first.

Most of us have had a car or truck. We're saying you've got a Ford car, let's put Ford parts in it. That's what the engineers developed them for. You wouldn't think about going to a Chevy dealer and putting a Chevy part into a Ford truck. You wouldn't think about putting the wrong part into the car because you know that eventually it will wear something else out and have more damage.

So when we test for and find a hormonal deficiency doesn't just make sense to replace those lost hormones with their bioidentical equivalent instead of a synthetic substitute?

Hormonal Balance and Ratios

The four principle sex hormones are both similar and different for men and woman.

- Hormones in Men: Testosterone, DHEA, DHT and Estradiol
- Hormones in Women: Estradiol, Progesterone, DHEA and Testosterone

We test for 4 major hormones for men and for women. Testosterone, DHEA, DHT, estradiol in men. Estradiol, progesterone, DHEA, testosterone for women.

Now, is the testosterone that we have here in men different then the testosterone that we have for women? No.

Are all these same hormones that are in men, the same as the hormones found in women? Yes. All of these that are found in women, are they found in men? Yes. So if these hormones are the architects that make up your body and you have the same hormones in male and female, why is it that we are different? Ratios!

The ratios are what make the difference. If you look to the man and you said "Wow! What a hunk!" you are actually saying "What a perfectly balanced ratio of hormones!" Well maybe not in so many words but let me explain.

The Statue of David, I always like to make that an example. You look at the statue of David and he is perfect. Perfect musculature, everything is perfect, perfect symmetry. If that statue of David had hormones and we check them, we'd find that his testosterone to estrogen ratio is 40 to 1.

Subsequently, we look at a beautiful woman with great skin, with great breasts, with good curves on her. Her estrogen to testosterone ratio would be the opposite. So it's not about what you have, but it's what you have in ratio to what else is on board. Is that confusing anybody? Let me try to simplify it.

Let's say you had a bus. In this bus we had 25 seats on the right and 25 seats on the left. On the right we had everybody wearing white shirts. On the left we had everybody wearing black shirts. As long as the number between them was 1 to 1, the white shirts and the black shirts were equal, the bus continues to go straight. IF someone in the white shirts get off, then all of a sudden because of the heavier amount of people on the left side of the bus, the bus would start to veer to the left. The more of the white shirts that get off, the more you veer to the left. Does that make sense? This is what is happening with hormones.

Now let's put it into perspective. A woman starts to make certain hormones and when she starts her menstrual cycle. What we call the sex hormones: estrogen, progesterone. When she is young and she's making these hormones, she makes a ton of them. So what happens to her breasts? From flat chested, all of a sudden her breasts start to come out. Why? Estrogen. Estrogen is supporting the function that tells the DNA in the breast tissue to start to develop. To start getting ready to be able conceive and subsequently to lactate. Then, after a certain amount of years of constantly making estrogen, what happens? The tissue itself starts to become less dense and they start to sag.

We have so many people that come in and they say, well that's gravity. It's not gravity. It has nothing to do with gravity. If the estrogen is there to support the tissue, the tissue will be dense.

When the estrogen is not there, the tissue becomes atrophied compared to when you were younger, all of a sudden the tissue is less dense and they start to deflate.

It's the same thing with skin. Skin starts to sag. Men have it also. Men start to sag.

Also, men start to develop breasts as we get older.

A twenty-two year old man came into the company one day. Visibly he was very distress and exclaimed, "I don't know if you can help me but if you can't help me I don't know what I'm going to do." He'd been to five doctors and no one could help him.

I took him under my wing and I tried to help him as much as I could because he really looked in bad shape. We checked his hormones and we found that his testosterone was 725. Now, the optimum levels for testosterone at the time were from 800 to 1,100 in men from the age 25 to 60 but the medically established level was from 230, (65 year olds) to 1,000 (25 year olds).

By the way, who do you think has got the 1,100? 25 year olds. Who do you think has the 800? The 40 year olds. I tell you this so you can start thinking in that vein.

Well he was 725, which is not really not that much lower than 800. So it doesn't encourage us to supplement with more testosterone. The real problem was that his estradiol, which is the strongest of all estrogens, estradiol was at 100. So it was a 7.25 to 1 ratio, instead of 40 to 1.

We checked his nutritional value and we found that he was very low in zinc. Zinc and raising his zinc levels, guess what happened? His testosterone went up, not very much, up to about 800. His estradiol went down to about 25. 800 to 25, which is a 40 to 1 ratio. All of a sudden his breasts start to atrophy and disappear.

Three months later he came again, into the company, and we talked. He said to me, "Do you remember when I told you I don't know what I'm going to do if you can't help me?" I said I did, and he continued, "I was contemplating suicide at the time. I didn't know it then but the estrogen that's in my body was getting me very, very depressed. The depression had me falling into almost suicidal tendencies."

I say to everybody, take a look at yourself right now. Put yourself in that mans place. 22 years old, you have breasts. Probably handsome at 17. So you can't take off your t-shirt, you can't play basketball with your friends, you can't go into a pool, you can't do anything . . . that's when depression sets in . . . I'm happy to say it was $2.98 a bottle of zinc that changed this guys life. Ultimately the zinc altered the hormones. It stopped the conversion of testosterone to estradiol. That gives you a little idea of what we're about.

It is not just replacing hormones. It is all about bringing your body into a natural hormonal balance. Once your hormones are balanced it is a lot easier to bring the rest of your life both physically and emotionally into balance.

We're not so much about continuously supplementing if you don't need it. What we want to do is we want to modulate the hormones. There are hormones in your body that are being changed right now. They're being changed by drinking coffee or soda, caffeine and sugar. Eventually these kinds of things exhaust the adrenal glands which produce hormones to help regulate energy. These are things that we are doing to ourselves and we don't know it.

I hope you're as excited as I am because I've changed my whole life based on what I have researched, practiced and shared about hormones. I feel that I have been able to help thousands of people.

Don't take our word as gospel on hormones. There are a lot of books, videos and resources on the internet to learn more about the role hormones play in our health and wellness. Be cautious though as you gather information. As I have mentioned, there is plenty of contradictory information about the synthetics vs. natural hormones generated by companies that have a vested interest in keeping physicians off track on the benefits on natural hormones and prescribing their brand of synthesized treatment.

Most doctors don't know about the stuff that I'm talking to you about. I spend half my time talking to patients and the other half consulting and educating doctors on this stuff. Really, we're learning from patients because the patients keep giving us more and more feedback. This is a very, very new science. You'll see it is very important.

DHEA

DHEA for a long time we didn't know what it was. It is the hormone that is most prevalent in the body. It is 80% of the hormones that are out there. But scientists didn't know what it was used for. They thought it was junk hormone, it's an intermediary hormone, it's a stepping stone in becoming something else.

But now we've found that DHEA may play a role in the treatment of certain diseases like fibromyalgia, systemic lupus and multiple sclerosis. That when we check these patients, that we find, not in all of them but in some of them, we find that their DHEA levels are suppressed. And guess what? When we bring their DHEA levels back up to normal they get better. And that's huge, because we're making a correlation, is it mind/body or is it body/mind.

Cortisol

Cortisol is increased with stress. It suppresses other hormones. The hormones that are suppressed build your body.

Here's something that no one ever told you, the human body is torn down and rebuilt over 90% of it over a 3 year period.

So, look at yourself. The person that you're looking at right now is not the same person that was here 3 years ago. Our cells have been changing. Your bones have been changing. Everything about you is changing.

Think of yourself as the ceiling. You're the ceiling tiles. Over a 3 year period somebody came in and took one tile today, next tile on Tuesday another tile from over here. Every day we walk into this room and you would think the ceiling was the ceiling. But over a 3 year period you've changed all the ceiling tiles. Would you notice? No you wouldn't. But that's what happening to you now.

You know when you really notice, when women goes into menopause either surgical or otherwise. When a man is castrated, all of a sudden their bodies change unbelievably. When we talk about hot flashes later, you will see that men can have hot flashes also, but only if they have complete testosterone suppression as in castration. Whereas women will have it without having complete estrogen suppression. Women have a higher chance of having more effects of hormones then men do because estrogen is a much stronger hormone.

DHT

What is DHT?

DHT is what is responsible for the solar panels that men start to get as they get older. On their heads, a little receding hairline that happens is dihydrotestosterone. It is the strongest of all the androgens. We want it, we need it and we need a certain amount of it to sustain an erection. Too much of it and all of a sudden now you start losing your hair. Guess what? When women come in and they have very, very fine hair and they have like where men lose it on either side, women will have this big part in the middle. That's also due to DHT.

Now, you may have DHT in a certain amount. Let's say, for arguments sake, and this is not the amounts that you have in your body, this is just a numerical factor for you to understand this. We have a DHT factor of 1. Your estrogen is a factor of 10. Well as long as 10 is going against 1, guess what happens? The bus leans toward the 10, you keep your hair. But now all of a sudden you have a very strong hormone, DHT, and instead of having 10 you have 1. Now all of a sudden the DHT is so strong it can show its face.

Did you ever see a maple leaf? You take a maple leaf in the summer time, you take it off the tree and you crumple it and you bring it back and it just pops right back into shape. Isn't that interesting? Now you take that same maple leaf in fall. Now it turns yellow, then it turns red then it turns brown. By the time it turns brown and you take that maple leaf and you crush it in your hands, you've got powder. You've all done it as kids, I'm sure. That red, that yellow, that brown were always in that maple leaf but you couldn't see it because the green was so strong it overpowered the other colors.

Just like when you were younger, your testosterone was so strong that you didn't see the estrogen inside of the man's body. Same thing with a woman. The estrogen was so strong the testosterone really didn't get a chance to show its face. As you get older, and older, and older, and you look at older woman, all of a sudden hair starts to spring out on their chin. Why? Testosterone is showing its face. Men start to develop breasts. Why? Estrogen starts to show its face. Now isn't it interesting that estrogen not only works on the receptor on the breast but also works on another place that men have estrogen receptors.

Now we usually have to be tested for it after we get above the age of 40. The prostate. As men start to get older, all of a sudden we need to have our prostrate tested. Why? Because testosterone starts to drop and estrogen starts to rise. The estrogen makes the breasts grow as well as makes the prostate grow.

Does this start to make a little bit of sense? Now you're starting to understand why things are happening the way they are.

Estradiol

Estradiol is the strongest of all estrogens. Just like testosterone makes a man a man, estradiol makes a woman a woman. Everything we find attractive about a woman, skin, hair, eyes, texture, breasts, wider hips, everything that's going towards procreation, has to do with estradiol. It is 10 times stronger than estrone and 100 times stronger than estriol. So, it is the female estrogen hormone. Regretfully the body has pathways in place to keep the estradiol/estrone ratio. Supplementing with just estradiol will increase your estrone ratio.

We check estradiol in men because we want to see that 40 to 1 ratio. If it's not we may ask you to supplement with zinc. If the DHT is too high, we may ask you to supplement with Saw Palmetto and bring it down, keep it in balance.

Estrogen

The BIG QUESTION, "Does estrogen cause cancer?"

Estrogen does not cause cancer.

It's like me saying does fire in a building burn the entire building down? If light a match in a building it will not bum down the whole building. The match has started something. It can be the catalyst to start something else. But letting the match burn itself out in an ashtray will do nothing to the building.

There are many different types of estrogen in your body. The three major ones are: estriol, estradiol and estrone. We call estrone E1 and it should be 10% or less floating around in your body. Estradiol E2 is 10% or less also. Estriol E3 is 80% or more.

Does estrogen cause cancer, no it doesn't. But Estrone (E1) when it gets metabolized, it gets metabolized to a particular hormone called the 16 hydroxy metabolite and the 2 hydroxy metabolite. That's the one that's geno toxic. That's the one that causes cancer. That's the one you start to make more and more and more of as you get older.

So the cards are stacked up against you. That's what happens. That's why when you're young the chances of cancer are negligible. As you age, the chances of cancer are higher and higher and higher.

Does that make sense? Think of it this way. Let's say this is one celled animals that we're talking about and these are the locks. These are now becoming the keys. X denotes bad hormones. Bad estrogen. O denotes good hormones. If we surround this cell with good hormones, the chances are that these good hormones will interlock with those receptor cites and the cell will stay normal. If we surround the cell with bad hormones chances are that these hormones will interlock with those receptor cites and the cancer risk will increase. Does that make sense?

If I said to you this thing is toxic, this thing causes cancer. Don't put it on your body. You would stay away from it. Regrettable, our bodies working against us, especially for women.

Progesterone

Progesterone is my favorite hormone. Progesterone is the feel good hormone. Guys when I tell you about progesterone, you're going to want to have a vat of it at home and the day that your wife gives you a hard time you're just going to pick her up and put her right into the thing like a dunking tank.

Now this is where the education really begins. Think about a person being on Valium. What do we think about when we see a person on Valium? The person is calm. The person is relaxed. In a calm voice they could say, "Oh, the house is on fire." that kind of thing.

Valium was made to interact with a certain receptor site in the brain called the GABA receptor cites of the brain. Guess what fits into that particular receptor site? Progesterone. Progesterone is there and works like the body's own Valium. That's why we call it the feel good hormone. You see, estrogen is much stronger as an anabolic hormone than testosterone. It causes the endometrial lining to get thicker, ready for implantation of a fertilized egg and it works quickly. It causes the breasts to get plump so that they'll be able to get ready for pregnancy. It does it quickly. It allows the skin to stretch. All of these things are done quickly. Why? It's a very strong hormone. Well, if you have a very strong hormone you need to have another counteracting hormone to quell the estrogen fire and that is one of progesterone's jobs.

How much does progesterone play a part in your lives today? Well, remember the news there was a lady that killed five children. Remember that. I don't know about you guys but I was screaming from the rooftops. Why was I screaming from the roof tops? Because when a woman gets pregnant the placenta starts to make progesterone. Think of this woman. She was neurotic, she was psychotic before she had gotten pregnant. She got pregnant and all of a sudden she was calm. Why? The placenta was making huge amounts of progesterone. How huge? Well think about it guys.

Let's take one of you guys. We'll have a volunteer . . . you're nice and healthy, we'll take him. We're going to put you on this table right here, we're going to cut him open and I'm going to stick my hands in there and keep pushing his guts around until I can fit one of those basketballs in there for 9 months. Volunteers? Any takers? That's what's happening. Woman are getting their guts just pushed out of the way but they don't feel anywhere near that type of discomfort had I done that to somebody. Why? Hormones.

So here we have this lady who is now high in progesterone she's taking care of one, two or three kids because she had 4 of them, 5 of them. Each time that she had a kid, all of a sudden she was a basket case again. So her husband said well lets get her pregnant again. He did it five times. After the 5th time, she wound up killing all 5 children. Think about what's happening.

Here she has this thing pushing her guts out of the way. And she's taking care of 4 children and she's still happy. How strong is progesterone? I'm telling you guys, you'll want a big vat of it at home so whenever you see your wife get really upset you pick her up, boom, put her right in. 1 know I have it, I have one wife, 4 daughters. I need 5 vats!

Estrogen

We call estrogen the gas in a car and we call progesterone the break. What you want to ride in is about 55 mph. But you need a certain amount of gas and at times you apply a little bit of break and you keep it at 55. What happens as you get older? The break goes away and little by little you've got a lot of estrogen and very little progesterone, comparatively. As the progesterone starts to drop, guess what? Your PMS, insomnia and headaches start to become more prevalent. Does it affect you only when you get older? No.

PMS. No such thing only PDS. Progesterone Deficiency Syndrome. The bloating, the irritability, the headaches, the cramping all have to do with not enough progesterone. Why? Because there's a lot of Xeno estrogens in the environment. False estrogen like compounds found in foods we consume, foods we give our children. Did you know estrogens are in compounds like plastic products? They are found in everyday things that we eat that will act in the body like estrogen. Look at a bottle of water. I'm just as guilty as everyone else. But I want you to start thinking. I want you to start thinking about where that bottle came from.

Filled with water they put it back out on the dock where the Arizona sun got to beat down on it. You ever go into a new car? You ever get a brand new plastic bottle and smell it? You can smell the petroleum product. Those petroleum products leach out into the atmosphere and leach into the water. Our brand new bottle of water that we drink has the most amount of petroleum products that it will ever have. What do we do? We drink it. After we drink it, do we save that bottle and say well a lot of the petroleum products leached out already and we'll fill it up with water again so we will not set more petroleum products into ourselves. No we throw it away and get a new one. This is common place, this is what we're doing in our society.

Anyone here on a diet? I always am dieting. Remember when you were younger? What did your parents say to you? Don't eat that candy because it's going to spoil your dinner. How many of us have a little piece of candy before we sit down to three helpings of mashed potatoes. Everybody right? You learned it from your parents. Your parents would never lie to you. They told you the truth. Did you realize that if you had just a little bit of candy, even rock candy or something, before you sat down to eat. Instead of getting real hungry and getting three scoops of mashed potatoes you'd get one and maybe eat that.

That's what's happening. This is something that we know. Just like the hormones, we know that we have them and their gone. If we could replace them, we'd be back to where we were before. We know that, we can inherently feel that. But what is the answer. The answer is the dieting with a little bit of candy and it doesn't hurt you. Not a lot. I didn't say to eat a box of candy . . . just one little piece of candy that will help in not eating 3 helping of mashed potatoes.

Testosterone

What is testosterone?

Testosterone is what makes a man a man. Everything that you feel that is manly has to do with testosterone. What's the difference between a 19 year old man and a 49 year old man? The 19 year old man goes out and plays basketball with his fellow fire fighters, sprains an ankle and 3 days later he's back on the court. The 49 year old fire fighter goes and plays basketball, sprains the same ankle, 3 weeks later he's still nursing it. What does it do . . . I'm not talking about the physical now, I'm not talking about what happens with his leg or his ankle what I'm talking about is what does it do to his head? Because 3 weeks later the guys go up to him and say hey you want to come out and play basketball? And he says no, I've got to bring the truck in for service. What he's really saying is not I can't risk hurting my leg again and he's making excuses and he's changing.

There is something that happens to men and women must be very sensitive to this because of all the things that are happening to them. You have to be sensitive to this because, believe me, I'm going to tell the guys how sensitive they must be to women because of all the things that are happening to them. You women have to be sensitive to what's happening to a man. There's a hormonal reason why the mid-life crisis happens. That hormonal reason is responsible for a man having 3 times more likelihood of committing suicide after the age of 50.

Nobody talks about it. Women talk about their hormone problems as soon as they start their period, or even before then. They're constantly talking about it. Men do not.

I can promise you there is no one here that stood up at the water cooler with the other fellow fire fighters or fellow men and said, "Hey, you know what, my erection isn't what it used to be." I guarantee it. Men don't talk about it. This is something that when we get our hormones back, you know what, it's going to change. Men are going to start feeling that we can repair hormones just like women have been repaired with hormone therapy for the longest time. We are going to encourage ourselves to get tested.

Women like to say that testosterone is a male hormone. But women have it also and the lack thereof there goes libido. I'm going to show you how, as your testosterone drops, your sex drive goes right down the drain.

Common Hormone Problems

The most common hormonal problem differs between males and females.

Common hormone problems for men include:
- Low sex drive
- Erectile dysfunction
- Enlarged prostate
- Weight gain
  - Especially in the middle of the gut
- Fatigue
- Irritability

All of these things are associated with low testosterone, low DHEA.

Common hormone problems for women include:
- Hot flashes
- Night sweats
- Insomnia
- Osteoporosis
- Low sex drive
- Irregular menstruation

Hormonal Decline With Age

The story of hormone decline. Men have this linear decline down to zero. Women have this bumpy road. Suddenly they get into menopause and boom. It declines quickly. Again, they talk throughout this whole time guys, you don't.

I love what happens with a young group of girls when one of them starts their period. It's very amazing. You'll see, I study this because this is my life, hormones are my life, they'll be in school and one girl has her period or at least the premenstrual part of it and she's doubled over by the wall and then there's another one here that's running interference for her. She's got her hand out—no one can bother her—she's not feeling well today. They're like guards, "You can't talk to her, talk to me. I'm taking care of her right now." They do that. When women get together, guys don't know this, and they become really close friends. Guess what happens to their period? They start to cycle together. How does that happen? How is it that the hormones that you have in your body start to assume the same properties that her hormones do? If you don't think that food and drink influences your hormones, you're very wrong.

Five of you will sit together and say I'll have salad, oh I'll have salad too, oh I'll have salad too. No one's going to say I'll have the double cheeseburger and pizza. It's not going to happen. You want to have wine? What kind of wine do you want? We'll try the red. Okay, we'll all drink the red. So we all drink the red, we all drink the white, we all have the salad, we all have the burgers. That's what you do.

Now extrapolate that even further. Look at a 90 year old couple. Here they are standing right in front of you. You get a good look at them. Their nose is the same size. Their ears are the same size. Their breasts are the same size. Their hips are the same size. Why? I have even gone as far as to looking at their arms and checking for age spots and they had the same amount of liver spots. Why? Because for 15 to 20 years they've sat across the same breakfast table, the same lunch table, the same dinner table, ingesting the same foods and letting the hormones from the food make them into the same person. They even think alike. Why?

Because they have the same hormones that are causing their bodies to be in the same fashion. They have very little hormone production on their own. 15 years of whatever they ate. You think they're going to make two different dishes for them? No. They make one you eat the same thing.

You don't believe me—think about it. You'll see that all of these things fall into place. All of these thing have a place . . . just no one has come out and said hey . . . this is what's happening.

Issues for Men

Men lose 2% of testosterone per year beginning in their late 20s. This can affect not only sex drive, but also energy levels, metabolism, weight and a whole host of other issues.

Some guys that eat healthy, vegetables, good food, organic beef and things like that still have a hard time losing weight. Guys that are doing the right exercises all the time sometimes don't lose much. Why is that? Hormones!

Even if you're trying to eat the right food, it doesn't necessarily mean that you're going to get the right nutrition. Society and environment factors themselves seem to be against us. One hundred years ago, 100 grams of spinach had 100 milligrams of iron. Today, 100 grams of spinach has 1 milligram of iron.

So I almost advocate to everybody over the age of 35 to be on some type of multi-vitamin. Because the food doesn't have it.

While men lose 2% of their testosterone per year, 1% is lost through testicular atrophy—as the testicles start to shrink they don't produce as much testosterone. The other 1 % is stolen by their blood system.

There are receptors in your cells that may act like keys to unlock the testosterone from the protein and make it available to the body's tissues.

We have what's called a steroid hormone binding globulin. This globulin actually pulls out the testosterone and once it gets its hands on it, it doesn't allow it to go into any of the locks.

Therefore fewer locks are being interacted with and the body is not being rebuilt in a younger fashion as it should be. So we start sliding down hill. Do the math. 25 lose 2% a year—a man at 50 is half the man he used to be at 25.

If we don't do the right things and we abuse our systems by eating fast food and by eating the wrong things and not taking the right vitamins, we are defeating ourselves.

Daily Testosterone Production

Testosterone, like many other recurring patterns in nature, tends to follow a biorhythmic cycle. As an example let's use a young male with no testosterone problems. At 11:00 at night he has starts to go through the high levels of testosterone and it peaks in the middle of the night as illustration use the number 10 as this peak. At 4:00 a.m. it starts to come down. Subsequently, when he's younger he'll wake up with an erection. That's because of the high amount of testosterone being made at night.

As he gets older, he starts losing that. Normally he gets another surge around 10:30 and he starts having another rise say up to a 7. It will give him an energy boost, gives him an urge to get going. Around 2:30—he's at the lowest. So a young man, this is the normal level, this is what happens throughout the day. No problem. Let's see what happens to a person as they get older.

As they get older, the same rhythm happens except his night peak is at a 2. Where's 2:30—down here at a zero. Look around the fire station, look around the nursing homes. Go there around 2:30. You're going to see two thing happening. Somebody with low testosterone will be sleeping; which is what happens in the nursing homes. You'll see all the old guys everybody is passed out around 2:30—its siesta time. Or they're heading for the coffee, chocolate bar, something to boost them up. Because their energy level is way down—they need the false energy sugar, something to give them a little boost to finish up the day.

Men benefit from restoring hormones to normal.

When they have:
Decreased sexual drive or activity
- Difficulty in achieving or sustaining an erection
- Weight gain or difficulty losing weight
- Decreased strength or muscle size
- Persistent fatigue
- Difficulty concentrating
- Mood fluctuations

So many guys come up to me and say I watch my weight. I went from 150 pounds when I was 25 to 150 pounds now that I'm 50. Except that the weight got redistributed. I used to be big in the chest and now I'm big in the abdomen. I don't know how it happened. Testosterone and Estrogen.

See guys say drinking beer gives you a beer belly. It's not a beer belly guys. The beer has alcohol. Alcohol converts your testosterone to estrogen. Estrogen then increase fat deposition. If I were to stop taking my hormones, my gut comes out. Even if I don't drink alcohol. I start taking hormones again, my gut shrinks. This is what's happening to us. You see a guy with a huge, distended gut and say well I drink a lot of beer. Well, it's not the beer. If s the beer that's causing your testosterone to become estrogen.

Well how about high estrogen, no progesterone. What do we have there? Psycho . . . a real psycho case. Anybody ever see a mean drunk? A mean guy who has a lot of testosterone in him. Big, burly type guy. He gets piss ant drunk and all of a sudden what happens to him? He's meaner than spit. Why? High amount of estrogen in his body, no progesterone. You slap progesterone on that puppy, he's coming right down.

Dr. Lee argues that you should have it in domestic cases. As soon as there is a domestic dispute, slap everyone with progesterone . . . doesn't matter who it is, calm them both right down. That's what will happen. Progesterone is the feel good hormone.

Guys, decrease muscle size, persistent fatigue, difficulty concentrating. This is the big one. Men have difficulty concentrating as they get older. Mood fluctuations. Varying things going on all the time. Alzheimer correlates with certain hormone levels.

Testosterone, it's just about survival. What happens to the man as he loses that testosterone? Well, when he was younger and he was all about testosterone, he'd make that house. My father says this about me all the time. You'd make that house if you didn't like the color. You'd burn it down to the ground and start it all over again. My father was the same way. All of a sudden in his 50s and his 60s that same guy that would make and destroy it because he didn't like the color, now he's yelling at me to shut off the lights. Are you going to be paying for that electricity. Because in his mind he's thinking, I have to work to pay for that electricity. When I was younger I could work all day and work all night and nothing bothered me. I was full of testosterone. Now I don't have it. I don't feel like working if I don't have to. So if s going to cost me for you to keep those lights on. Better yet let's let sunlight come in. Have some sun domes installed so we don't use any light at all. That's what's happening. I could tell you a couple stories about my dad.

The first one I could tell you about is I remember when he was younger, remember this is in the Bronx, there was a lot of fires in the Bronx, and I said dad there's a car outside and it's on fire. He looked at me and said it is your car? I was 9 years old. Of course it's not my car. Don't you want to see? If it's not your car, don't worry about it. Mind your own business. Then he turned 63 and he's standing outside, I went to visit him at his house, he's by the gate. I said, what's up dad? He said ifs around 3 p.m. a dog does his business right on that fire hydrant and then I have to go outside and clean it up. The guy who couldn't care less if outside his house there was a car burning when he was younger, now all of a sudden is worried about dog poop next to the fire hydrant on the street. Why? Lack of testosterone.

Testosterone as a Cancer diagnostic: We recently had a patient that was put on the hormone combination high in testosterone. After a few days he started to get pain and discomfort in his groin area. He went to the doctor that told him get off the testosterone. They did tests and found out he had prostate cancer. His doctor said that had he not been on the testosterone they may have never caught the cancer until it was too late. The use of the testosterone allowed to grow from the size of a pea to the size of 2 peas quickly and this caused pain. Had he not used it, the cancer may have silently grown to the size of a grapefruit without any signs over time.

I recently talked to a patient that had been taking injections for testosterone and complained that his level had never increased over 236 in the blood. So he was always tired and felt terrible. So I told him about the PLO Gel we make and he got his physician's approval. We started him on the gel. In a short time, his level was 1100 and we had to back him off a little and he felt great. His PSA also went up. His doctor said he wanted to take him off. He asked the doctor is there any way that he could stay on it. The doctor said I'm scared that you might have cancer and I could not let you stay on it unless we had a biopsy of the prostrate. He said do it, I don't want to get off this stuff.

Issues for Women

Hormones effect women in a more dramatic way during menopause and perimenopause. What is perimenopause? Perimenopause can last up to 10 years before she goes into menopause. So the person you married 20 years ago is not the person you're going to be living with for those 10 years. It is not going to be perfect. Believe me.

Do you want to know the real truth about it? What did I tell you happens to a person that has a lot of estrogen and low progesterone. Irritable. The women that we were just talking about. As you get older . . . you make a certain amount of estrogen . . . the follicle will start making a certain amount of estrogen and it makes the corresponding amount of progesterone. So when you're younger it makes a high amount of estrogen, a high amount of progesterone. As you get older, unenthusiastic volunteers, you get less estrogen and less progesterone. But now all of a sudden the fat cells start taking over the job and making more estrogen compared to progesterone. Remember we talked about this. So now, we make more estrogen. Where's the balancing part of the progesterone. Who's making that? Nobody. So you become irritable, you can't sleep at night, these things start high amount of headaches, high amount of estrogen. Everything that we consider someone the "B" word, to make a long story short, is because of high amount of estrogen, low progesterone. So even though it is less estrogen than we started with, it is much more.

Now, we'll think back to people that are really irritating you and you'll say, you know what, she does have high estrogen signs compared to her progesterone. She talks to everybody about how she doesn't sleep, she talks about how irritable she is, how things just set her off and things like that. High estrogen, low progesterone.

Hot Flashes

Have you ever had a hot flash? Do you know what a hot flash is? For the guys, you really don't experience hot flashes unless you have been medically castrated or something to that effect.

What a hot flash is like you're walking along and all of a sudden you're in a 200 degree dome. You take another couple of steps you're down to 40 degrees. You take another couple of steps you're back at 200 degrees. How well can you function? Not very well. Most people become basket cases.

Think about it. 50 hot flashes a day for about 5 to 10 years, how would you handle it? Not good. Guys I'm talking about this because you need to be sensitive to what's happening to our women. The minute you understand what's happening to them, it's easier for you to help them or at least be supportive. It's easier for you to get together, it's easier for you to live together.

Night Sweats

Night sweats are the same thing. Except it's when you lay down, because the blood is shunted into different places all of a sudden the whole body becomes profusely hot and you start wetting the bed. Not because you urinated on the bed but we have children that come to us and say mommy was in bed and all of a sudden I felt as if she wet the bed.

Well, let's say I took one of you put you here. I took one of your children and put them in the other room. Then I put a heavy weight on your foot that you could not get off. It would hurt like hell. What are you going to do? You're going to scream for your child and he doesn't come to help. How's the next call going to be? Louder, stronger, more forceful. You're going to give it everything you have. Well, that's what's happening.

When you first started your period, the body sent a message from the brain called follicle stimulating hormone to the ovary and said I need a volunteer and 16,000 volunteers died that day in the very beginning. You have 400,000 follicles. 16,000 died that very first day. Subsequently less each month. But I ask you this question. I need a volunteer. Come on somebody, anybody. She volunteers, she volunteers we get them both out of the room. Ask for another volunteer. I guarantee you when I said the word volunteer somebody looked down and said please don't pick me. Usually the guys in the back by the way.

But now think of the ovary. Every month it asks for volunteers and they're taken out. Then it asks for more volunteers and takes them out. Eventually whose left, the guy that was in the back that when I first said volunteer looked down and said I don't want to be one. How well is that volunteer going to make estrogen? How well is that volunteer going to make progesterone? Not very well. So how much of these hormones will it make. Not very much. What happens to your breasts? They start to sag. What happens to your skin? It starts to sag. Do you see a trend of what's happening here?

Think about 20, 30, 40 years passing of menstruating. What's going to happen to your body? Who's left to make the estrogen? Not too many enthusiastic ones. Then what happens? Guess what? The body's smart. The body's real smart. The body says we need estrogen and we don't have it. Is there any other organ out there that can help us?

I got it! The fat cells. The fat cells can make estrogen. Well too bad it only makes the bad estrogen, but I need estrogen so we're going to have to take whatever we can get. So estrogen makes fat cells larger, which makes more estrogen, which makes fat cells larger, and there's your answer to why when you were young you could eat anything you wanted and now you just look down the Twinkie aisle and hips start popping out. Estrogen enlarge fat cells.

Insomnia

Think about a person that's on Valium for a long period of time and now we take them off of it. Think they're going to sleep? Nope. Think they're going to become insomniacs? Yep. Not enough progesterone or Vitamin D.

Osteoporosis

Think of the Pac Man game. We have two cells, two different types of cells inside the bone. One is called an osteoclast, it eats up bone. The other is called osteoblast, it actually makes more bone. The osteoclast that eats up bone is slowed down when you have the right amount of estrogen. The osteoblast that makes more bone is sped up when you have the right amount of progesterone. So progesterone is actually helping you increase bone.

We have great drugs out there for people who have osteoporosis. Fosamax, Actonel, Miacalcin all of them increase bone density 4-6% over 24-36 month period. It's not bad. You're slowly dropping bone, but all of a sudden you're increasing 4-6%. That's not a bad deal. But when you get the hormones right, you can increase bone density by 18-22% over the same amount of time. Naturally with those hormones that make bone.

Low Sex Drive

Low sex drive is a big problem. Oprah had a show 3 to 4 million woman in this country don't want to have sex anymore while they're still married to their husbands. Why? Testosterone deficiency. In essence what happens is the fat cells are making estrogen. They just don't magically make estrogen. What they do is they take the testosterone and they change it to estrogen. That's why as the testosterone level starts to drop, so does the libido start to drop.

I once had a woman come in and say to me "I don't want to have sex anymore. I'm 65 and I feel we should be done with that by now. My husband says he still wants to, that horn-dog, and he's 70. So I'm here to check my hormones."

We get her on the program and four months or so went by before I saw her again. I asked her how she was doing, knowing perfectly well she was doing well. Her make-up was done, her hair was done and she had a smile from ear to ear. She went on to say "I'm fine what are you going to do about my husband?" He had gone from a horn-dog to impotent in 3 months, just because she felt better.

We had one patient who was 41 years old and one of her complaints was that in her 41 years had never had an orgasm. She had had several relationships but the Big O had eluded her.

We recommended balancing her testosterone which we did. Later I received a phone call and she exclaimed. "There's life down there!" She had her first orgasm at 41. She asked me could it be that I have been having hormonal problems all my life and that conventional medicine never picked it up. I said there is a good chance that is exactly what happened.

The stories are endless. I was recently at a Christmas party and a woman comes up to me and says are you Rudy? I answered yes and she yell out "Honey, this is the guy that helped me with my hormones!" and a man from across the room full of people yells, "Hey Rudy, thank you for the best sex I've ever had!"

Recently I read an article calling estradiol the strongest of all estrogens. The love hormone. Estradiol the hormone that allows us to love which makes sense. Women fall in love when they are young and fall hard. But men, when they are young can be ruthless because they have small amounts of estradiol. The older we get the more men have, which allows men to have mature relationships and get married, and the less that women have which allows them to settle for less than prince charming.

I remember a woman coming in and telling me that her insurance will be no longer active and she would have to pay for her hormones out of pocket. I told her that it would be about $60.00 per month for the formula. She got on her cell phone and told her husband. The next time she came in she said that her husband understood $600.00 a month and that he would entertain getting a second job so she would be able to afford it.

Irregular Menstruation

This is a big one. Young people, when you have a young person turns 15, you give them a driver's license. A driver's license allows them to drive. Conventional wisdom says that if you have irregular menstruation the doctors will now give you a birth control pill. What do we give our children when we give them a birth control pill? A driver's license allows them to drive. So a birth control pill gives the consent to do what? Don't do that.

All girls, if they have irregular menstruation, or when they do have irregular menstruation, often it's because of the food we consume. The fast food, the junk food and everything else we eat is heading you down that road.

When they have a problem, they should be tested and they should be supplemented with natural hormones, we should replace what is no longer there because of what we did as a society or what we did as parents in raising them.

I told my wife, it's our fault. We have to be able to sit there and say no to birth control pill, let's give them whatever it is necessary for them to grow up naturally.

Most of the time, it is simply the lack progesterone that leads to irregular menstruation cycles.

Poly Cystic Ovary Disease (PCOD)

A patient walks into the pharmacy with classic symptoms of poly cystic ovary disease. She had broad shoulders, a distended gut, a full beard that she had to shave twice a day and was at a loss of how to proceed. Her testosterone was very high and needed to increase her female sex hormones. After getting her hormones in balance and three months of therapy, I witnessed a new person walk thru the door. She was there to pick up her prescription. She was at the front counter when I walked out from the back room. Immediately her eyes flooded with tears. She said she couldn't thank us enough and how she tells everyone about us. Seventy percent of the hair on her face had fallen off, her shoulders had narrowed, her distended gut had reduced greatly and she had started to regain her womanly features.

Hormonal Changes

All anti-aging protocol says that if you want to mess around with a person's hormones and you want to make them feel better you want to bring their hormones up to the top 1 /3 of the normal range. So the more we bring back the hormones to the top-1/3 of normal—the higher probability that these people will have their bodies rebuilt in a younger fashion.

In a typical perimenopausal person, her estrogen, progesterone and testosterone all drop. Now the fat cells take over the job to make more estrogen. So where do we go? We go up higher in estrogen, not into the normal ranges, just so that now it dominates over the progesterone. So we have a scenario, which we call the dominating scenario, where estrogen is dominating over the progesterone and you still don't have enough estrogen. So you have estrogen overdose effects without having even enough estrogen. Headaches and still having hot flashes. Estrogen effects without having enough estrogen.

So here you have a person that is going to be very irritable and not much sleep. Then what happens as this estrogen continues to go up, the testosterone goes down, down, down, down, down. What we're saying is, we know what's missing, you're telling us the symptoms, and we're going to give you that hormone. Once the symptom is alleviated, we've reached a mark. If it hasn't been alleviated we'll keep giving you more until we reach that mark. First we balance to the right ratio. Then we worry about increasing you to the right level.

Everybody's different. Look around you. If I said to you today I'm going to give you four sizes of shoes a one, a four, an eight and a fourteen. Who's going to be happy here? Probably nobody. You go back to the doctor and the doctor says, we gave you this hormone, and you say, but doctor I still don't feel like myself. Well here's some Prozac. One, two punch. Here's the horses urine, it doesn't work for you, here's the Prozac. One or the other is going to have to help you. It's true. That's what is happening across the country right now.

How much can hormones affect a person's mood? I remember one day a woman came in and asked for her prescription saying she had been off of everything for weeks. She went to the front counter. She picked up a snickers bar and got frustrated because she could not open it. BAM! She threw it at me and hit me right in the face. I quietly picked it up, peeled it like a banana and gave it back to her. She left crying. Her husband came in later and picked up her prescriptions. Days later she came back and apologized.

How much does this affect the partners life. The pharmacy closes at 6:00 p.m. It was Friday and at that time we were closed the weekends. A man came in at five minutes to six with an empty bottle of his wife's custom hormone capsules. I looked at the record and said to him that she was early. She should have enough at home. He exclaimed that she usually transfers a weeks' worth to her purse but he was in a panic he said. I cannot go through the weekend without them. I'll give you $200.00 to stay late and make them. That's how much of a difference it was making in their lives.

Perimenopause

What is perimenopause?
- Hormones begin to be out of balance
- Irregular cycles, emotional and mood changes
- Ovaries begin to stop producing eggs
- Can last up to 10 years

Perimenopause can last up to ten years. Hormones begin to be out of balance. Your regular cycle, emotional, mood changes, ovaries begin to stop producing eggs.

So you go to the doctor. The doctor says we have a drug called Premarin to balance out your hormones. It comes from pregnant mare's urine. It says so right in the name . . . <u>PRE</u>gnant-<u>MAR</u>es'-ur<u>IN</u>e . . . PRE-MAR-IN . . . Premarin.

Don't believe me, crush the tablet, put it in warm water put off to the side, go visit it in three days. It'll smell like a latrine. That's what we're giving our mothers. That's what we're giving our wives and sisters. They are synthetics. If you're supplementing with synthetics your chances of cancer are higher.

When a women's hormone levels start to drop as in perimenopause, the body's defense mechanism is to allow fat cells to convert testosterone to estrogen. The ovary was making estrogen and the corresponding balanced amount of progesterone because of the extra estrogen. The pt will become estrogen dominant with estrogen dominant symptoms and yet not have enough estrogen. For example, let's say that the normal level for progesterone and estrogen is 100 for both figuratively speaking and in deficiency the patient makes 50 and 50. Now the fat cells kick in and increase the estrogen to 75 and the progesterone stays 50. Eating soy will fool the body into thinking that it has 125 of estrogen and the liver will remove 25 to bring it into the level of 100. But what it really did was to bring the body's own estrogen back down to 50 and balance of with the progesterone. The overall effect of keeping the estrogen at a much lower level is that the body will decrease the formation of secondary female characteristics such as smaller breasts will be seen. Over a long period of time (3 years) and the benefits of against osteoporosis and the other degenerative diseases will be lost.

Menopause

What Is Menopause?
- Ovaries stop producing eggs
- Levels of estrogen, progesterone and testosterone fluctuate
- No menstrual period for 12 months

What are the symptoms and causes?
- Hot flashes = Low estrogen
- Memory loss = Low estrogen and low progesterone
- Night sweats = Low estrogen
- Mood swings = Low progesterone
- Vaginal dryness = Low estrogen, low progesterone and low testosterone
- Sleeplessness = Low progesterone
- Painful Intercourse = Low testosterone

These are just some of the symptoms, but you don't have to live this way!

Guys, think about this . . . not enough estrogen, not enough testosterone, the wall of the vagina becomes very thin. As it becomes thin, it allows blood vessels to move to the forefront. As that happens, there's a higher degree of UTI-urinary tract infections and intercourse becomes painful. The truth is if intercourse is painful, nobody, with the exception of the masochists, would want to have intercourse. Nobody would! So you have to be sensitive.

When we're talking about progesterone and I'll get my wife involved in this one. She's a constant case study for me. I have a constant way of being able to adjust her. I'm going to throw you three little stories that happened with her because I think it will really exemplify the reality of this.

We we're moving a big couch. As we were moving this big couch she goes, "Ouch . . . oooh my period came."

I say, "Why? What's the matter? Isn't it supposed to come?"

"Yea . . ."

"Are you late or anything?"

"No . . ."

"So what's the problem?"

"I didn't get any cramping. I didn't get any bloating. I didn't get any headaches."

I tell her, "I hate to tell you this, you're on the hormones now, and you're not supposed to get cramping, bloating and headaches. You never were supposed to get it."

She says "But if those don't happen, how are you going to know your period is coming so you don't have an accident?"

It's funny because I remember one time she says to me, I'm sitting there watching television, there I am with my remote, typical testosterone male. Ladies as soon as you have more testosterone, you start manipulating the remote. Just to let you know. So here I am clicking the thing. She comes by and says isn't it hot in here? The thermostat is on the wall, I can see it and it says 70 degrees.

I said, "Well hun you've been running after the kids, put on the air conditioner." About 20 minutes goes by and here she comes, "Isn't it cold in here?" I go, look at the thermostat its 70 degrees. "Well honey put on the heat." After a while I sat down with her and I said, "Hun it's not hot or cold in . . ." here pointing to the room, "but it's hot or cold in here," pointing at her.

The more you understand about hormones when you're younger the better it'll be. If I had my choice I would ask everybody, when they're feeling their best, to take all the tests, see where all your hormones are and then when you don't feel well, 10, 20, 30 years from now revisit those tests. Whatever's missing put it back. Because that's what's gone. That is what makes sense. But nobody does it.

I'll give you another one. Anybody here ever have a chocolate craving? Sweet craving. When men have chocolate craving or sweets craving it's usually due to low magnesium. If we give you magnesium, within 20 minutes of taking a capsule, your chocolate craving is gone.

When women have a chocolate craving it's a life or death situation. I was hoping you ladies would laugh. But you know it's true. Do you want to know why if s true? If I said to you we have a person in front of us and they're going into diabetic shock—too much insulin. Is that a life or death situation?

Do you want to know why it's true? If I said to you we have a person in front of us is going into diabetic shock, what's happening with that person? Their blood sugar is going down and it could send them into a coma.

When estrogen is dominant, perimenopausal, remember dominant doesn't have to be high just higher than the progesterone the yeast in your body starts to flourish. When the yeast in your body starts to flourish the yeast sucks out the sugar from the blood. As it sucks out the sugar from the blood, what happens to the sugar in the blood? It plummets. So your brain says, "I'm dying, I need sugar." Just as if you were a diabetic patient, when estrogen is dominant, your mind changes it to, "I want a double-dutch chocolate sundae."

Now for the guys out here, how many women have had that double-dutch chocolate sundae and the minute they finish with the double-dutch chocolate sundae say, "How could you have let me eat this?"

One day, before we adjusted her, my wife walked into the kitchen and said, "Leave me alone. My period is coming and I'm going to open the five pound Hershey bar."

So I said to her, "Calm down" . . . what's the message? Ooh the Hershey bar. I saw in her eyes that if I didn't get out of the way I was going to get hurt.

So I said hold it. You know I talk about this let me prove it to you. I took 100 milligrams of progesterone, it is in a cream, and I put it on her body. I took a teaspoon of sugar and I said let that dissolve under your tongue. Ten minutes, just sit there. If in 10 minutes if you still want it, I'll give you the Hershey bar. I'm sitting there guarding it in the kitchen. I'm sitting in the kitchen, every once in while I look out and she's sitting there, nice and quite watching TV. About 10 minutes pass—nothing. She doesn't come in and ask for it. Fifteen, 20 minutes pass. Finally I pick up the Hershey bar and I go over to her. I say, "Honey do you want it?" She says "Oh please, I couldn't even look at that." I said, BAM, I've got something.

Once you've finished that double-dutch chocolate sundae or whatever sugar may be around, you have 2,000 calories sitting in your gut, only 100 calories went into the blood stream and saturated the craving. Eventually those 2,000 calories will deposit somewhere. Then you'll be real angry about it. Women have more willpower then men until their hormones are out of balance, then they are at their mercy.

We did a little study ourselves. We took women in their 40s and we found that 95% of them have low or below normal estrogen readings. 86% of them had low progesterone or had low normal progesterone. So here we are. We go into the 50s and what do we find? 80% had low estrogen readings and 94 of them had low progesterone readings.

What's happening? If that little cell, that egg cell, is responsible for making the estrogen and the progesterone, it would follow suit that in their 40s that if 95 percent of them had low estrogen readings and 86 percent of them had low normal progesterone readings, and the progesterone went down even further in their 50s, you think the estrogen would go down too. But it doesn't. Why? Because the fat cells start making more estrogen. Do you see what's happening? That's the proof of the pudding. That's why we know that the fat cells are making more estrogen.

Synthetic Hormones

- Increase the risk of cancer
- Contain estrogens and progestins that are foreign to the body
- Some use chemicals and pregnant mare's urine, as a base
- Can cause undue weight gain, skin allergies and other side effects

Herbal Remedies

- No testing available determine individual needs
- No cardiac or osteoporosis protection
- Hit-or-miss on hormone levels needed
- No follow-up consultation to assess results

FlashX, Ridaflash, Dongquai, Evening Primrose all of these things, that are advertised as being helpful for menopause. They are good as band-aids. They are good to help reduce the hot flashes in the short term.

What you want to do is you want to replace the right estrogen to get your body back into balance. Help osteoporosis. That's the whole thing. Our slogan is "Return to yourself—return to who you want to be. We all can think of a time when we ourselves felt more energetic, more like the people that we always thought we would always be. Then all of a sudden for whatever reason, as age comes on, we start losing that little by little.

Benefits of Natural Hormone Therapy

- Relieve symptoms of PMS, including bloating, cramping and irritability
- Relieve migraine headaches
- Promote healthy bones
- Restore a healthy sex drive
- Decrease fatigue
- Relieve depression
- Migraine headaches
- Topical creams avoid kidney and liver
- Bio-identical" (human-identical) hormones—exactly like the hormones produced naturally by our body
- Bio-Identical" hormones are made from vegetable sources
- Custom formulated by a compounding pharmacist

Balanced natural bio-identical hormones are essential to health and wellbeing. There are millions of people that don't know about this, they are learning, little by little. Many doctors either don't know or have been misinformed about the benefits and proper use of bioidentical hormones. That's why I spend so much time trying to make healthcare professionals understand. They don't teach this in medical school. They don't. Dr. Lee will tell you "I wish they taught me this in medical school". We should be taught conventional and natural naturopathic ways.

One patient that came in pale as a ghost and said to me "Call my doctor and get me some of that progesterone."

"Well, no." I said. "We're supposed to test you, see if your levels are low and then recommend . . ."

"Oh my God. Call my doctor." she insisted.

I call the doctor and okay, here's the progesterone. I'll authorize the prescription said the doctor. I told him we have to test . . . he says, give her the prescription that you think she should be on based on your experience. Okay, I made one up, 100 milligram dose, I said this is the same dose that I would use for my wife with a chocolate craving, I'm sure this is going to be able to take the edge off of the estrogen dominance. I gave it to her. She went into the bathroom and applied it. She sat in front of me. I'm doing my work and there's a little chair right there and she's sitting there. About 20 minutes pass, her headache subsided and color came back to her face . . . what happens if it wears off and the headache comes back she said. I said here's the prescription this is how much you need.

I said to her, when you have symptoms, call me and I'll keep telling you what to re-dose yourself with until you, yourself start saying 1 know exactly what I need to make myself feel better. Because it's not all the time it's just a certain period during the month. Usually a week or so before the period when that usually happens. A lot of people say I'm dying of cancer or something, my head, no one else in the world can have this kind of pain. Many people do. You are more common than you think. Regretfully, doctors don't know about it. We're trying to get the word out.

More benefits of natural hormones. Typical creams reduce the amount that is cleaned by the kidney and liver by 80 to 90% that of an oral dose. Bio-identical-human identical. Hormones exactly like the hormones produced naturally by your body. Bio-identical hormones are made from vegetable sources custom formulated by a compounding pharmacist. That's me and the crew.

The Natural Solution to Hormones

- Test, don't guess
- Supplement to balance hormone levels if low or low normal (vitamins & hormones)
- Use only all-natural vegetable sources for hormones
- Prescription formulations custom-made by hand to your test results

When it comes to hormones, test—don't guess. Don't go into the store and say I need DHEA because I have fibromyalgia and buy the DHEA off the shelf. Don't buy the progesterone that's over the counter. Why? Because if you overdose yourself with the progesterone you will push other hormones down. We have something that's called hormonal tension. Something that's called hormonal load. These are words I've made up because they are not in the dictionary. I'll explain to you what these mean.

Hormonal tension means that if I give you a certain hormone, I will suppress a corresponding hormone. We have a patient that has polycystic ovary disease. She's a woman that looks like a male truck driver stereotype. What you would call a bearded lady. Full beard. She comes in, we give her a certain amount of estrogen, a certain amount of progesterone, at a certain level, we push down her testosterone. We push down her DHEA which were at astronomical levels. Higher than what a man would have. Guess what happens? The hair on the face falls off. The hips start to increase. The gut shrinks. The breasts start to come out. She becomes more womanly. Why? 90 percent of your body is rebuilt over a three year period. It is constantly being rebuilt. With the right hormone therapy you can get rid of bad hormones. Guess what happens? The body starts to replace itself in the right way. That's hormonal tension. Hormone affecting the levels of other hormones.

Let's say you had a body with only 4 hormones. Hormonal load is the certain amount of hormones total the body will allow in it. When you push it beyond that level, it starts getting rid of them. It tells the liver to start getting rid of them. So let's say I went to the health food store and bought DHEA. I took my DHEA and I took the wrong dose and it went real high. Since this one is so high, the body starts cutting them down and cutting them down, and cutting them down. What happens to three of them? They're non-existent. What happens to the thing that had to be rebuilt by those three. They're not going to be built in the right fashion. So, doing it on your own is a big no no. You need to be tested, you need to be listened to by a professional that knows what the symptoms are and slowly tweak. It's pretty much like taking a square peg and trying to put it in the round hole. You shave a little here, you shave a little there and you keep shaving at it until you fit it in.

Think about it. When you went for a wedding dress or for the guys, if you've gone for a custom made suit. My father was a tailor. You'd go once, twice, three times for a fitting until it gets right. Because you need it for your body.

What Does a Compounding Pharmacist Do?

- Serves as the link between the patient and doctor
- Custom makes the cream or capsule hormone supplements
- Works with both patient and doctor to cure symptoms

What do we do? We as compounding pharmacists, we act as an intermediate between patient and the doctor. The doctor will see your results; the doctor will give you a prescription we review it and custom make the hormone supplements tailored to your specific needs. We have you rechecked and make adjustments to help get your hormones corrected and maintain hormonal balance throughout your life.

Take the 18 symptoms, headaches, irritability and all those things. Put down a number 1-10.

Example: How important is that insomnia? It's a 10 . . . You can't sleep at all at night. So we start you on a certain amount of progesterone and all of a sudden you sleep 5, 6, 7 hours.

A lady came in and said to the other pharmacist, "May God bless you."

I said "Why?"
"I had the first 6 hours sleep in I can't remember how long."
It's a big deal. So now she's getting sleep. So now it's not a 10 anymore it's a 5 or a 4. The more you keep telling us what you're feeling the better we know how to treat you. The big word is, COMPLAIN. You must complain. It's the only way we can get to feel your best. The biggest enemy to feeling great is feeling good. If

you feel good you won't strive to feel great. If you keep complaining to us we'll keep helping you and tweaking it, and tweaking it, and tweaking it until you get the product you're happy with.

A Heritage of Hope, Help & Healing

Hope, help and healing, this to me is a goal that I've set out for myself. I've set it out for a couple of different reasons.

I was at a karaoke place with my 9 year old daughter many years ago. We're sitting there and a lady with obvious polycystic ovary disease is there. Due to imbalance in her hormones she looked more like a man than a woman. I looked at her then said to my daughter, "I can help her . . . I need to talk to her. But how do you go to this stranger in a t-shirt and shorts and tell her, 'Lady I can help you?'" My daughter said, "Do it dad." I went back and forth and finally I just went over to her and said here's my card, my name is Rudy Dragone I think I can help you. She said, "I've been to so many doctors and no one can help me." I told her to take the test, I'll pay for it. My daughter looks at me when I return to the table and says, "You know dad? You're an angel because she was praying and God sent you to help her." I stood there thinking I don't consider myself to be an angel, if anything I consider myself a sinner. I'm not a holy person, but in this respect I looked at my daughter and my daughter is looking at me like I looked at my dad. I've got to do this. I've got to keep telling people there is hope, there is help.

A few years back my father had a heart attack. I went back to visit him in New York and they put a stent in his heart. After they put the stent in his heart about 8 months later I told my dad, come on out, spend time with the family. He said "I can't." I said why not?

"Because my heart hurts."

I said okay. Back to New York and I'm sitting there with a cardiologist and a radiologist and we're looking at his heart in an angiogram. They said, "See these arteries here in the heart? They're all diseased. So we're going to have to cut here, cut here, cut here and we're going to do a bypass." I said "Whoa, time out, what are you talking about here? Are you talking about open heart bypass surgery?" the doc said yes, "If you don't he's going to die. No if, ands or buts, he's going to die." I sat there and I said, "No my father's got hemochromatosis, diabetes poor circulation and he's got osteoporosis." But, like any other dad he doesn't listen to his son when I told him I could help him. Now that changed. So the doctors said to me, "This is what we have to do. If you take your father out of here his life is in your hands." So I went to my dad. I said dad, this and this and this is what they're saying. My father looked at me from the table and he said, "My mother died at 24 giving birth to my brother, my father died at 58, I'm 65 maybe it's my turn to go." I said "Well if you think it's your turn to go I'm going to call Bellevue and I'm going to have them come pick you up because you're crazy. You should be kicking and screaming." Everybody should. Nobody should want to die.

I said, come back with me to Arizona and we started him on all sorts of vitamins. We got his insulin need down from 100 units a day to 40 units a day. We started him walking, very, very slowly at first. The man would only walk 2 blocks and get chest pains. We started him on hormone therapy for testosterone that increases the blood flow to the heart in patients that have heart problems by 68%. AMA study, not mine, the AMA says it works. Not only does it do that but the effects were shown even 33 months after discontinuing of the hormone therapy. Not like nitroglycerine that works for a certain amount of time then it's gone. So we started him on testosterone, DHEA, pregnenolone. We got all of his hormones back up to a youthful level. I got all of his vitamin levels back up to a youthful level. Got him on chelation, remember I was talking about alternative therapy.

We hit him with everything in my arsenal. The man that couldn't walk 2 blocks without having chest pains, my dad and I went hiking up a local mountain. Three quarters the way up, he looked at me and he said "I can make it to the top." He had broken his leg once and he said, "I won't go up to the top because I'm scared that if I fall and break something you're going to have to carry me down. But my heart can make it!" We came back down from the mountain and we're sitting in the car and he's going back and forth with his hands. I said, "Pop what's the matter." He said, "Thank you for saving my life." I started to cry.

I've done great with my wife, I've done great with my children but nothing was important to me as my father saying to me thank you for saving my life. Because of this, I cannot keep my mouth shut. Because of this, I have to go in front of you and let you know about this stuff and don't take my word for it.

There are books out there. Go to the internet. Go to other doctors. Go to naturopaths. Go to wherever you have to go to get as much information as you can. Sometimes honestly, you'll learn something that we didn't know. There's no way we can read every book out there. You'll come up to us and say, well what do you think of this? Then we have to study that so as to find out what it is.

I ask you, I beg you, please go out there and learn as much as you can about this because it really can change your life and the health and wellbeing of those you love. It has in my family.

—Rudy Dragone

Clinical Reference Guide
Bioidentical Hormone
Replacement Therapy

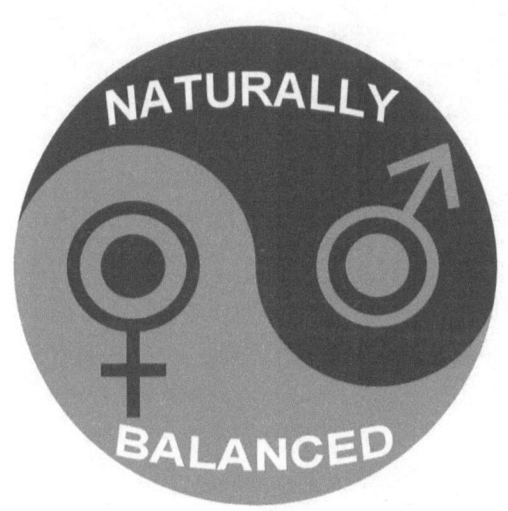

Symptom Worksheet
For Hormone Imbalance
or Deficiency

If you are experiencing any of the following symptoms, you may have a hormonal imbalance or deficiency. If left untreated, a hormone imbalance can cause serious medical conditions.

Please indicate on a scale of 1-10, with 10 being the most severe, any symptoms you are experiencing.

Rating	Woman	Rating	Men
	Irritability		Thinning Hair On Beard
	Fatigue		Thinning Hair Over Body
	Depression		Low Sexual Drive
	Headaches		Disturbed Sleep
	Hot Flashes		Depression
	Night Sweats		Prostate Enlargement
	Forgetfulness		Muscle Weakness
	Weight Gain		Fatigue
	Insomnia		Irritability
	Joint Pain / Backache		Thinning Skin
	Palpitations		Slow Wound Healing
	Crying Spells		Poor Concentration / Memory Lapses
	Loss of Bladder Control		Abdominal Weight Gain
	Burning or Pain Upon Urination		Loss of Interest in Surroundings
	Vaginal Dryness		Night Sweats
	Low Sexual Drive		Loss of Bladder Control
	Decreased Sexual Activity		Palpitations

	Loss or Thinning of Hair		Insomnia	
	Other, Please Explain on Back		Other, Please Explain on Back	

Additional Information:

For Women		For Men	
Date of Last Pap Smear:		Date of Last PSA Exam:	
Date of Last Mammogram:		Date of Last Prostate Exam:	
Date of Last Period:			
Number of Days in Monthly Cycle:			

Please PRINT Name:_____

Signature:_____Date:_____

Please feel free to fax me at 480-575-0541 or email me at Rudy@ ClarksPharmacyAZ.com for a free evaluation. Thanks, Rudy!

Clinical Reference Guide

- Who has hormone deficiencies?
    - Men: Due to the steady decrease of approximately 2% per year of testosterone after the age of 25-1% due to Sex Hormone Binding Globulin (SHBG) and 1% to testicular atrophy
    - Women:
        - Irregular menstrual cycles in the young
        - Perimenopausal patient
        - Surgical menopausal and other
- What is optimal hormone level? Top 1/3 of "normal limits" for good hormones and very little for bad.
- What's the order of priority in hormone testing?
    - Thyroid
    - Sex Hormones (balancing)(vitamins)

- o Adrenals (replacement)
- o Growth Hormone
- o Others (Pregnenolone)
- How are hormones replaced? Safely stay within the physiological levels whenever possible EXCEPT FOR: PCOS and anovulatory cycle.
- What problems occur with hormone therapies when giving melatonin and GH? When a patient has a cortisol deficiency, these will aggravate hormone deficiency.
- What problems occur with hormone therapies when giving thyroid therapy?
  - o Cortisol deficiency increases by increasing cortisol catabolism
  - o Decrease in cortisol will increase the change of the T4 to T3 and precipitate a hyperthyroid incident (this occurs more frequently under stressful conditions).
  - o Estradiol (E2) deficiency-low E2 causes an increase in the conversion of T4 to T3.
  - o Thyroid deficiency aggravates thyroid deficiency by decreasing the conversion of T4 to T3
- What problems occur with hormone therapies when giving cortisol therapy?
  - o DHEA deficiency—cortisol treatment suppresses adrenal function thereby decreasing ACTH and DHEA.
  - o Aldosterone deficiency—cortisol will decrease ACTH, which will decrease aldosterone.
  - o DHEA will decrease cortisol production by decreasing ACTH.
  - o Fludrocortisone will decrease ACTH, which will decrease cortisol.
- Why is Estradiol (E2) elevated in a progesterone deficiency? Because Progesterone (P4) helps change E2 to Estrone (El), which then converts to Estriol (E3), therefore of P4 is low, E2 will raise b/c the conversion from E2 to El and El to E3 won't occur.

- Why elevate Estradiol (E2) in a thyroid deficiency? Because it increases Thyroxine Binding Globulin (TBG) and decreases the conversion for T4 to T3.
- Why elevate Estradiol (E2) in a testosterone deficiency? Because it increases Sex Hormone Binding Globulin (SHBG) and blocks androgen receptors.
- Why does elevated progesterone aggravate aldosterone deficiency? Because progesterone blocks the aldosterone receptors in the kidney.
- Testosterone therapy with Estradiol (E2) deficiency causes what? An increase in the conversion of Estradiol (E2).
- What's the preferred route of administration for the following hormones;
  o Melatonin—SL
  o GH—SQ
  o Thyroid—PO
  o Calcitonin—Nasal
  o Cortisol—PO
  o DHEA—PO/SL
  o Estradiol—Transdermal
  o Progesterone—Vaginal/PO
  o Testosterone—Transdermal
- What are the dietary effects of a Paleolithic Diet? Good proteins such as meat, fish, poultry and eggs increases: GH, Cortisol, DHEA, E2, P4 and testosterone, however, bad proteins, i.e., milk products, decrease the aforementioned hormones.
- Saturated fats do what? Increase GH, Cortisol, DHEA, E2, P4 and testosterone.
- What's the net effect of Hormone TX on other hormones?
  o Melatonin
    ▪ Increases: GH, Thyroid, IGF-1 and insulin
    ▪ Decreases: Cortisol, E2, P4 and Testosterone
  o DHEA Increases: GH, Thyroid, IGF-1, Insulin, E2 and Testosterone
  o GH Increases: Melatonin, Thyroid, IGF-1, E2, P4 and Testosterone and Decreases: Cortisol

- o IGF-1 Increases: GH, Thyroid, Insulin, E2, P4 and Testosterone
- o T3/T4 Increases: GH, 1GF-1, Insulin, E2, P4 and DHEA and Decreases: Melatonin
- o Insulin Increases: Thyroid, IGF-1, E2, P4 and Testosterone
- o Estradiol (E2) Increases: Melatonin, OH, IGF-1, Insulin and P4
- o Testosterone Increases: GH, Thyroid, Cortisol, DHEA, igf-1 and Insulin
- o Progesterone (P4) Increases: Gil and IGF-1
- Progesterone can decrease the levels of what in both males and females? Estradiol (E2)
- What are the sliding effects of hormones?
  - o Pregnenolone & Progesterone—Low P4 causes decreased pregnenolone, which increases short term memory loss, therefore, increasing P4 & Pregnenolone causes pregnenolone to stay as pregnenolone, short term memory comes back.
  - o P4 & Testosterone—some patients taking P4 causes an elevation of testosterone causing acne in females.
  - o Testosterone & Estradiol (E2)—patients with low Zinc increase Estradiol (E2) when taking testosterone.
  - o DHEA & Testosterone-
    - If the patient has a low DHEA: give DHEA, which will increase both DHEA and Testosterone
    - If the patient has elevated testosterone and low DHEA: give DHEA, which will increase both DHEA and Testosterone; 3. If too much DHEA is given: DHEA will increase and Testosterone will decrease.
  - o P4 & E2—if small amounts of P4 are given, E2 stays OK; if too much P4 is given, E2 decreases
- What is a poor man's thyroid test? Basal Metabolic temperature for 10 days

- What is hormonal tension? Some hormones affect other hormones in the same category,.i.e., if we give Estriol (E3) only Estradiol (E2) increases.
- What are signs of hormonal deficiencies?
  - Melatonin—lack of sleep—TX: 0.5 mg to 5 mg SL AVOID: nicotine, caffeine, and alcohol.
  - GH—sagging face—DC: L-Arginine 2,000 mg and L-Glutamine 2,000 mg PO with dinner have them fast for 12 hours and sleep 8 hours during the 12hours of fasting—this will increase GH by 700%, depending on how low the levels are.
  - Additional Signs of Hormonal Deficiencies

Complaints	Physical Signs
ENT Infections Weight Gain/ Obesity Fatigue	Puffy
Brittle Nail Growth	Overweight
Intolerance to Cold Dry Hair	Dry thick brittle hair
Dry Skin	Diffuse hair loss
Headaches	Loss of outer 1/3 of eyebrow
Bloated Abdomen Tinnitus	Swollen eyelids, lips, tongue
Constipation	Abnormal sized thyroid (goiter)
Morning Hoarseness	Dry, rough, scaly skin
Muscle Joint Pain/Stiffness	Cold, swollen hands
Slowness/Sluggishness	Yellow palms
Apathy Dyspnea	Thick swollen calves
	Non-pitting edema of LE's
Morning Depression	Cold flat feet
Slow Thinking	Yellow soles
Easily Distracted	Bradycardia
Poor Concentration	Sluggish deep tendon reflexes
Poor Attention	
Poor Memory	

Lab Tests	Optimal Values
TSH	1
Free T3	3
Free T4	1.5
ATG	0
ATPO	0
TSI	0
Thyroglobulin	<10

2 types of TX for hypothyroidism: i. T3 10-75 mcg QID (fast onset and short duration-3-4 h) and ii. T3 SR 50-300 mcg QD or BID (slower onset and longer duration 1-8 h)

**NOTE: T4 has slower onset to activity, up to 10 days, it is less effective than medication containing T3. **

BEST OPTION: Desiccated thyroid (Nature's Thyroid) 1/4 grain to 5 grain tabs. FDA Guidelines: 38 mcg T4 9 mcg T3 allow 9 mcg slide; Nature's Thyroid only 2 mcg slide.

HOW TO SWITCH: 100 mcg T4 =1 grain Nature's Thyroid

Strong thyroid stimulators are: GH, IGF-1, and TEST

Mild thyroid stimulators are: DHEA, Androstenedione, and Progesterone

Strong thyroid inhibitors are: oral Estrogens and Cortisol at high doses

Mild thyroid inhibitors are: Transdermal estrogens and cortisol at physiological doses

What conditions can increase the need for thyroids? Winter, high altitude, high physical activity, high protein diet, low caloric diet, low veggies, oral vitamin E, lack of sleep.

What conditions can decrease the need for thyroids? Summer, living near the sea, low stress, high veggie diet, low protein diet, high caloric intake, untreated cortisol deficiency, testosterone in females, GH and insulin.

d. What's seen in someone with cortisol deficiency as a child? Thin, narrow body, high ENT infections, GI troubles, difficulty eating, high attraction to sugar.

Complaints of Cortisol Deficiency	Physical Signs of Cortisol Deficiency
Anxiety	Thin
Depression	Obese if sugar is craved
Moodiness	Hair loss w/ elongated hair root
Stressful situations	Brownish face
Decreased memory during stress	Hollow cheeks
Excessive sensitivity	Painful sinus
Feeling of being a victim	Enflamed/Red ENT
Paranoid	Swollen abdomen
Emotional	Brown elbow, armpit, hand folds
Yelling	Wet hands and feet
	May have high temp during follicular phase
	Wheezing if asthmatic
	Tachycardia
	Hypotension
	Painful muscle and joints
	Painful spleen upon palpation
	Sluggish deep tendon reflexes

Hydrocortisone Replacement	
Sedentary	**High Stress**
Female: 15 mg-40 mg QD	1.5-3x the normal dose
Male: 20 mg-60 mg QD	
Divided over 2-4 per day	

**NOTE: With Cortisol TX ALWAYS make sure the patient has appropriate anabolics on board. **
**NOTE: Naturally increase cortisol, increase light, small frequent meals, Paleolithic diet, avoid stress. **
Strong stimulators of cortisol: Test, DHT, Anabolics, mild thyroid
Strong suppressors of cortisol: GH, high thyroid and melatonin
Mild suppressors of cortisol: oral estrogens, DHEA and fludrocortisones

**REMEMBER: USE HIGH DOSAGES UNDER STRESSFUL CONDITIONS AND LOW DOSAGES UNDER UNSTRESSFUL CONDITIONS!!!

IN THE EVENT OF AN OVERDOSE: DECREASE THE DOSE BUT DO NOT ELIMINATE

**REMEMBER: Cortisol partially blocks the conversion of T4 to T3

**TROUBLESHOOTING:
- Swollen face (all day and night)—Too much cortisol
- Swollen hands and feet—High salt intake
- Puffy face only in the morning—Possible thyroid deficiency
- Too much cortisol—Ovary is agitated, insomnia, bruising, thin skin
- High sugar will decrease cortisol production
- GI problems may occur while on therapy due to decrease mucosal production
- Low B/P may occur while on therapy due to changes in aldosterone

"Wilson's rT3 Thyroid Syndrome"

- Wilson's Thyroid Syndrome' describes a population of patients who have normal thyroid blood tests (TSH/T4), and yet experience symptoms of low thyroid and low daytime oral temperatures. (< 97.8').
- Low average daytime oral temperatures (<97.8)
- Frequent history of childbirth, fasting, dieting, or high stress, causing impaired peripheral thyroid metabolism. Can be associated with high cortisol and malnutrition (low albumin, low selenium)
- Presumably (> Low T3/rT3 ratio)
- Dr. Denis Wilson popularized the use of T3-sustained release.

THE GOAL IS TO TX THESE PTS SO THEIR TEMP COMES BACK TO NORMAL AND THEY FEEL BETFER.
WILSONS ARGUMENT IS THAT THE LOWER A PATIENTS TEMPERATURE, THE LESS FUNCTIONAL ARE THE ENZYMES. HE SAYS THE ENZYMES SLOW DOWN DUE TO CHANGING SHAPE THRU CURLING UP FROM LOW ENERGY.

** SEE THE SEPARATE WORD DOCUMENT BELOW ON "T3 PROTOCOL" REVISED **

- Patients with low daytime temperatures and 'hypothyroid' symptoms may respond to T3 therapy.
- Order T3 Starter Pack:
  - 7.5, 15, 22.5, 30 mcg sustained-release T3 x 20 each.
  - plus 37.5, 45 mcg x 14 each (if necessary)
- Rx: start w lowest dose T3, give every 12 hours, each day progressing to next higher dose, etc.
- Baseline oral daytime temperatures
- Gradual increase in dosage, every 1-2 days
- Stop dose increases if:
  - Temperature goes up to normal or
  - Symptoms improve significantly or
  - No change in symptoms or temperature even after going up in dose to 60 mcg ql2h
- Rx:~30 days at that dose, q12h
- Reduce dose if:
  - Aggravations occur, such as racy heart, insomnia.
  - Give "test dose" of T4 12.5mcg to stabilize the T3, this commonly calms down the blood level fluctuations.
    - If it fails to stop the aggravation then you really are at too high a dose of T3 and go down

WHEN SX'S GET BETTER AND I FIND TEMPERATURE GETS BETTER, YOU STOP AT THAT LEVEL UNTIL NO FURTHER IMPROVEMENT FOR AWHILE

IF PT MAKES IT ALL THE WAY UP TO 60MCG Q12H W/O ANY IMPROVEMENT, THEN NEED TO WEAN THEM DOWN AND APPROACH THE CASE FROM A DIFFERENT ANGLE AS ONE OR MORE OBSTACLES TO CURE ARE STILL PRESENT. MAYBE IT'S LIVER, MAYBE NUTRIENTS, MAYBE SOMETHING ELSE.

- Unstable or rapid T3 metabolism sometimes causes racy symptoms while taking T3
- A test dose of T4 (125 mcg) is given when an aggravation occurs.
- If the symptoms are caused by T3 instability, the symptoms will typically resolve within 20 minutes of test dose.
- Patient then resumes the T3 protocols as before.
- If symptoms not resolved, patient is instructed to reduce T3 dose.
  - o Recycle T3 back down.
  - o Reduce dose in opposite direction, every other day.
  - o After reach dose discontinuation, stay off of T3 completely for—4 days, then
  - o Repeat cycle back up again as before.
    - As a rule, the dose required to produce an effect gets lower each cycle.

Goal: To produce sustained improvement and increased temperatures without dependence Rx T3.

PATIENTS WILL HATE YOU FOR REDUCING THEM OFF OF THE T3 BUT IF IT WORKED THEN THEIR T3 LEVELS WILL BE FINE AS THEIR THYROID AND METABOLISM HAS RESET SO THEY DON'T NEED THE T3 SUPPLEMENTATION ANYMORE. YOU MUST USE THE NUTRITION, DIET, AND HERBS TO ENABLE "THE BEST SUCCESS POSSIBLE FOR THIS TX.

OFTEN AT THE END OF THE 2ND OR 3RD ROUND, USUALLY ON ABOUT THE 3RD DAY, THE THYROID KICKS BACK INTO FUNCTION AND SEE TEMP COME BACK TO NORMAL WHERE-UPON THEY ARE NOW DONE W/TX.

Naturopathic "Wilson's"

To improve T4 to T3 metabolism, correct treat the cause:
- Mind-Body, stress, Life-style
  - Modulate cortisol rhythms
  - Diet, exercise, sleep
- Nutritional support
  - Selenium, Zinc
  - B12, Antioxidants
  - EFAs
- Herbal support:
  - Withania, Guggul, Ginseng, Bacopa

T3 THERAPY INSTRUCTION SHEET

1. Please take temperature every three hours, three times per day at the times indicated and record them on the temperature log (on back). Average these three temperatures each day by adding them together and dividing by three. Enter this average in the Average column on the log.
2. Take dosages as indicated according to the schedule/ temperature log (over).
   a. Notice that your prescription of T3 (starter pack) comes in various dose strengths
      i. e. 7.5 mcg, 15.0 mcg, 22.5mcg, etc., in multiples of 7.5.
      ii. You will also notice several "test doses" of 14, 12 mcg each, to be used only as directed, in case of symptom aggravation. (explained below, Item C)
   b. Starting with a 7.5 mcg dose of T3, you will be taking one dose two times per day, every twelve hours, i.e. 8 AM, 8 PM.
      i. Try to take the doses as close to this twelve-hour schedule as possible.

c. You may increase to the next higher level (+7.5 mcg) each day (see log), provided the average temperature remains below 98.0 orally.

d. Please note that you may combine capsules of different dose-strengths to add up to one dose of a higher strength,

    i. e. 45.0 mcg dose = 37.5 mcg +7.5 mcg (you may use two or more capsules to add up to your desired dosage)

3. Continue increasing the dosage by 7.5 meg each day until one of the following happens:

a. **If your average temperatures have come up to normal (above 98.0)**, or if you find relief of symptoms with significant improvement in overall well-being, you may stay at that dosage without increasing further.

    i. If temperatures then drop again you may resume increasing doses to the next higher level. If temperatures stabilize you will be prescribed T3 at that dosage.

    ii. Contact your physician regarding a prescription at the appropriate dosage level, and for instructions relating to duration of this treatment dose and when to cycle down again.

    iii. It is generally recommended that one maintain this dose level for about one month before cycling down, (read instructions for cycling down).

b. If the symptoms are not much improved and **the average temperature remains below 98.0** orally, continue to increase the dosage each day as directed.

    i. If there continues to be no significant change in your temperature or your symptoms, you may continue to increase the dosage by these scheduled intervals until you have reached levels of 60 mcg twice per day.

      ii.   Unless otherwise directed by your physician, we generally recommend that your dose not exceed 60 mcg every twelve hours.

           1.   At this point it would be recommended that you cycle down gradually. (read directions for cycling down).

  c. **If you begin to feel hyper, racy**, or if you can't sleep due to over-stimulation or speedy sensations in your body, you may be experiencing instability in T3 levels (rapid metabolism) or overdose in T3 medication.

      i.   We recommend that you take one dose of the T4 (12 mcg) "test dose". If symptoms are relieved within about 20 minutes, this is suggestive of T3 instability.

      ii.   In this case, we recommend that you continue to increase the T3 dose on the prescribed schedule. If symptoms are not relieved at that point, it is generally recommended that you decrease your dosage by 7.5 mcg each day until this symptom is alleviated.

      iii.   After this you may be asked to cycle down (see instructions below) or maintain the lower dosage for a longer period of time.

      iv. You will need to consult your physician for specific guidelines on your protocol in this situation.

4. **CYCLING DOWN**: T3 therapy generally includes a protocol we call cycling. Your physician will instruct you when it is time to cycle down. At that point you will gradually lower your dose in the reverse order of the way you increased. Your dosage will go down (by-7.5 mcg) to the next lower level every other day until you have gone completely off the medication. Wait at least three days before resuming T3 therapy. Unless your symptoms are much improved and/or your temperature has become normal, you will then be asked to cycle back up again_ Cycling up involves the same directions as when you first began T3 therapy. It's simply like starting over. We generally find that the dose required to

produce effective results gets lower each time one cycles up and down again_ You may be asked to cycle up and down in this fashion several times to produce the desired effect This is part of the strategy for restoring normal function without medication. With effective therapy symptoms will resolve, temperatures increase, and/or even the lowest level doses will not be tolerated without a feeling of over stimulation.

5. Please call office if you have any questions or problems.
6. Kindly give four days' notice for any necessary prescription refills.
7. If for any reason the medication is to be discontinued, the medication should not be stopped abruptly, but should be decreased gradually.

T3 THERAPY

PATIENT NAME: _____

DATE	DAY #	A.M. DOSE	P.M. DOSE	TEMP10AM	TEMP1PM	TEMP4PM	NOTES
	1						
	2						
	3						
	4						
	5						
	6						
	7						
	8						
	9						
	10						
	11						
	12						
	13						
	14						
	15						
	16						
	17						
	18						
	19						
	20						
	21						
	22						
	23						
	24						
	25						
	26						
	27						
	28						
	29						
	30						
	31						

COMMENTS:

Algorithm for Women

Menopausal
- <u>Low Everything</u>
- <u>Low Something</u>

Supplement to top 1/3 of luteal recommendations Middle of the road for menopausal is:
- <u>Except for estrone, we want that as low as possible</u>
- <u>Progesterone 100 mg-200 mg</u>
- <u>Blest 2.5 mg or Estriol 5 mg-10 mg if patient has a history or family history of cancer</u>
- <u>Testosterone 2.5 mg</u>
- <u>DHEA 5 mg</u>

These are "middle of the road", therefore, start here and adjust as needed

Non-Menopausal or Perimenopausal
- Estriol 5 mg-10 mg on days 5-28 of menstrual cycle **AND**
- Progesterone 100 mg-200 mg days 5-28 of menstrual cycle **OR**
- Progesterone 50 mg days 5-13 of menstrual cycle and 100 mg days 14-28 of menstrual cycle

<u>**Symptoms that should correlate with test results:**</u>

- Irritability—low progesterone usually a week to 10 days prior to the start of the period, they will say, "I don't feel like myself."
- Fatigue—low testosterone, also check thyroid levels, i.e., TSH, T3 and T4.

REMEMBER—thyroid levels may be deceiving; they were originated by taking a sample of people that had thyroid problems, therefore, inherently; lab results will be scheduled to the lower range.

**Ask patient to take basal metabolic temperature every morning for ten (10) days. Normal axillary and oral temperatures are 97.6 and 98.6 degrees Fahrenheit, respectively.

****Regulate** by using **Nature Thyroid** 16.25 mg daily and increase by 16.25 mg every 11 days until basal morning temperature is between 98 and 98.6 degrees Fahrenheit, accordingly, i.e., axillary and oral, respectively or the TSH is between 1.0 and 1.5.

**Fatigue can also be adrenals, therefore, check cortisol and DHEA *levels—Regulate* by targeting the top 1/3 of the normal range (laboratory dependent).

- Depression—most often due to low progesterone, also consider low thyroid levels. **REMEMBER**: Progesterone binds to the GABA receptors of the brain, exactly like Diazepam (Valium). Must have vitamin D above 50 for this to happen.
- Headaches—most often due to anabolic dominance. If the headache is behind the right eye, this indicates left brain testosterone dominance—check for acne and/or anger. If the headache is behind the left eye, this indicates right brain estrogen dominance—check for irrational and/or irritability.

NOTE: It is important to note that dominance can happen even with low levels, in other words, even if a patient has low estrogen, but progesterone is even lower, there can be estrogen dominance, therefore, check estrogen:progesterone ratio.

- Night sweats, hot flashes are surges of FSH and LH—happen for three reasons:
  - Not enough estrogen
  - Too much progesterone
  - Change of estrogen either up or down too quickly
- Forgetfulness—low progesterone. When the body has maintained a low level of progesterone for a long period of time, it compensates by converting pregnenolone to progesterone; when this happens short term memory suffers many patients can replace pregnenolone,

however, it is better to replace progesterone and pregnenolone together.

NOTE: By replacing progesterone alone you will know you are at the correct dose when the short term memory comes back due to NO conversion of pregnenolone.**

- Weight gain—estrogen dominance causes sugar cravings; responsible for 5-12 pounds of excess water. Check thyroid for hypothyroidism and adrenals!!!
- Insomnia—low progesterone use half hour before bed time (HS) to give calming effect. The target should be 7-8 hours of sleep with NO residual sleepiness (drowsiness). **REMEMBER:** As one increases the progesterone, increase the Blest, somewhat, but NOT at 1:1 ratio, because of the ratio staying the same.
- Joint pain—look for DHEA deficiency, i.e., SLE (Lupus), fibromyalgia, MS, and other connective tissue problems.

NOTE: 80% of the patients with these disease states have low DHEA, therefore, when the DHEA is replaced, the symptoms tend to disappear. **

- Palpitations—caused by elevated thyroid activity (hyperthyroidism), increasing thyroid hormone too quickly, estrogen dominance or low progesterone.
- Crying spells—low progesterone. **REMEMBER**: As a woman a goes further into perimenopause and/or menopause, the fat cells will compensate by making estrogen, however, there's no compensatory system for progesterone, hence the patient ends up with low estrogen as well as estrogen dominance.

NOTE: Fat cells do not make estrogen from "thin air" they convert testosterone to estrogen. *

- Loss of bladder control—loss of testosterone over time leads to lose of sphincter and muscle integrity.
- Vaginal dryness—low estrogen and low testosterone.
- Low sexual desire—low testosterone.

- Testosterone 2% cream: place rice size amount applied to clitoris and nipples one hour prior to coitus.
- L-Arginine 1,000 mg-1,500 mg orally: one hour prior to coitus to increase chance of orgasm.
- Decreased sexual activity—low testosterone and low estrogen leads to increased vaginal atrophy causing painful intercourse.
- Estriol 1 mg via vagina: at hour of sleep for 14 days then 2-3 times per week. This will rectify the problem until the topical hormone levels are normalized.
- Loss and/or thinning of hair—elevated DHT compensated by elevated estrogen.

NOTE: In Perimenopausal women, we must first align the thyroid and adrenals. When the thyroid is not up to par, the body will believe it is starving so that hormone binding globulin will increase in the blood and attach to steroid hormone keeping them from binding to the receptor. The blood test may show normal hormones are there; however, they may be bound and inactive.

TROUBLE SHOOTING

While a patient is on hormone treatment, as a rule of thumb, if the hormone isn't achieving the needed result, double the initial dose; if this "new" dose is too much, split the difference of the increase, eg., initial progesterone dose is 100 mg and we've established it's too low, increase the dose to 200 mg (double), if we then determine it is too high a dose, then split the difference (100/2 = 50) and the new dose is 150 mg. If this new dose is not enough, split the difference again (50/2 = 25) and the newer dose would be 175 mg.

NOTE: This is done ONLY if the patient considers the problem a "10' on a scale of 0-10, otherwise, leave the patient on the same dose for 60-90 days; this is so because it takes that long for the receptor sites and new hormonal signature to develop.

- We must listen to the patients, therefore, increasing and decreasing dosages accordingly. Most patients will have overly excitable receptor sites and over time will calm

down, needing lower dosages initially and more over time.
- Thyroid function devastates hormone balance.
- In the event of high stress, i.e., death in the family, it may be necessary to double the dose for 1-2 months.
- 11% of thyroid patients have iodine deficiency and not "thyroid problems".
- If a patient has normal T4 and low T3, think of adding Bromine supplements to the regimen.
- BE ALERT: When treating a couple and the male is on testosterone supplementation and the female partner has elevated testosterone levels, think cross contamination.
- Change one hormone at a time to remove "10's" from the symptom chart (0-10 rating).

Saw Palmetto—stops testosterone from becoming DHT
Chrysin—helps test from becoming DHT
Progesterone—helps test from becoming DHT
Zn—prevents test from becoming estrogen
DIM—allows estrogen to go down "safe" pathway, i.e., estradiol to Estriol

Generalities

Body Type	Male	Body Type	Female
Ectomorph	Norm	Ectomorph	Low Estrogen, Progesterone and Testosterone
Mesomorph	Norm to Low Testosterone	Mesomorph/"Hour Glass" Shaped	Normal Pattern
Endomorph	Low Testosterone/ High Cortisol	Endomorph	High Cortisol
		"Pear" Shaped	High Estrone and Low Progesterone
		"Large Breasted" w/ Small Hips	High Estradiol and Low Progesterone

Algorithm for Men

Symptoms that should correlate with test results:

- Thinning of hair on beard and/or body—low testosterone
- Depression—low testosterone, consider decreased thyroid activity
- Disturbed sleep—low testosterone
- Prostate enlargement—elevated estrogen to testosterone ratio; elevated estrogen
- Muscle weakness—low testosterone
- Fatigue—low testosterone, consider decreased thyroid activity
- Irritability—low testosterone, high estrogen
- Thinning skin—low DHEA.
- Slow wound healing—low testosterone; consider diabetes mellitus, check HgB A1c
- Poor concentration and/or memory lapses—low pregnenolone, check atherosclerosis
- Abdominal weight gain—elevated estrogen and low testosterone; consider metabolic syndrome, check HgB A1c
- Loss of interest in sexuality—low testosterone
- Night sweats—very low testosterone (testosterone fatigue failure)
- Loss of bladder control—low testosterone
- Palpitations—low testosterone, consider increased thyroid activity
- Insomnia—low testosterone

NOTE: Due to the steady decrease of approximately 2% per year of testosterone after the age of 25, all that is needed 90% of the time is to supplement according to the deficiency of testosterone.

NOTE: The "cocktail" is complemented with:

- Progesterone 4 mg to keep the testosterone from becoming DHT or E2.

- DHEA according to the deficiency to keep the testosterone as testosterone and not lose it due to high DHEA
- Chrysin and DIM to maintain the conversion down the "safe pathways"
- Zinc 100 mg and at least Copper 3 mg per day to decrease estrogen formation in men

NOTE: Progesterone in men above 10 mg per day may cause loss of erection.

TROUBLE SHOOTING

- While a patient is on hormone treatment, as a rule of thumb, if the hormone isn't achieving the needed result, double the initial dose; if this "new" dose is too much, split the difference of the increase, eg., initial testosterone dose is 100 mg and we've established it's too low, increase the dose to 200 mg (double), if we then determine it is too high a dose, then split the difference (100/2 = 50) and the new dose is 150 mg. If this new dose is not enough, split the difference again (50/2 = 25) and the new dose would be 175 mg.
- We must listen to the patients, therefore, increasing and decreasing dosages accordingly. Most patients will have overly excitable receptor sites and over time will calm down, needing lower dosages initially and more over time.
- Thyroid function devastates hormone balance.
- In the event of high stress, i.e., death in the family, it may be necessary to double the dose for 1-2 months.
- + 11% of thyroid patients have iodine deficiency and not "thyroid problems".
- If a patient has normal T4 and low 13, think of adding Bromine supplements to the regimen.
- BE ALERT: When treating a couple and the male is on testosterone supplementation and the female

partner has elevated testosterone levels, think cross contamination.

- Change one hormone at a time to remove "10's" from the symptom chart (0-10 rating).
- L-Arginine 1,000 mg to 1,500 mg orally: one hour prior to coitus to increase chance of orgasm—may combine with Viagra or other ED medication.

Signs of Low Testosterone in Men	
Pale	Male pattern baldness
Slumped	Undeveloped beard
Fragile	Dry eyes
Kyphosis	Dec. axillary and pubic hair
Lordosis	Gynecomastia
Obesity	Hemorrhoids
Cellulite	Poor concentration
Nervous	Poor memory
Depressed	Weak heart beat
BPH	Decreased musculature
Decreased testicular size	Decreased size and girth of penis
	Peyronie's Disease

**NOTE: DHT is used for Peyronie's disease 25 mg/ml, apply 1 ml on "curve side" of penis daily; or to counteract gynecomastia. **
**NOTE: Usual Testosterone dose: 50 mg/ml to 300 mg/m1-1-2 ml QD **

When is Testosterone Lowered or Raised?	
Increase Testosterone with:	**Decrease Testosterone with:**
Low protein diet	High protein diet
High fiber diet	High fat diet
Low calorie diet	High calorie diet
Increased physical activity	Decreased physical activity
Chronic stress	Unstressed vacation
Diarrhea	
Progesterone TX	

NOTE: <u>Testosterone doesn't cause cancer!**</u> It's decline and **preponderance** of estrogen causes cancer, therefore, use testosterone to our benefit by knowing if the cancer is presents quicker. **

- Increased estrogen in men is caused by what? A. caffeinated drinks, B. alcohol, C. wearing tight underwear, D. obesity.
- How do we intervene? A. Zinc 100 mg QD, B. Progesterone 5 mg QD, C. Anastrozole 0.5 TIW or BIW or QW x 30 days.
- To lower estrogen and Sex Hormone Binding Globulin (SHBG):
  o Decrease alcohol intake
  o Decrease caffeine intake
  o Increase nitrogen balance (high protein)
  o Decrease obesity
  o Use loose underwear and pants
- High fat and aromatase changes testosterone to what? Estrogen
- What is varicocele? Testicular blood stagnation
- How is it cured? DHT onto vein or surgery
- Too much testosterone can cause what? Elevated estrogen
- Therefore, do what? Lower testosterone
- Too much thyroid causes what? Increased change of testosterone to estrogen

- Therefore, do what? Lower thyroid
- Decreasing GH will do what to aromatase activity? It will increase it.
- Therefore causing what? Elevated estrogen
- The lower the testosterone and DHT in a person, the aromatase activity? Higher
- Cortisol deficiency leads to what? Testicular insufficiency
- Which does what to Sex Hormone Binding Globulin (SHBG)? Increases it.
- Which does what to androgen activity? Decreases it.
- Which increases what? Aromatase
- Which in turn leads to what? Increased estrogen.
- Progesterone deficiency decreases the conversion of what? Estradiol (E2) to Estrone (El) to Estriol (E3)
- Foods that decrease estrogen effects and estrogen are what? A. meat, B. soy products, C. carotene vegetables, D. shellfish, E. reservatrol, F. vitamin C and K, G. zinc, H. niacin
- RX's that decrease estrogen include what? A. spirinolactone, B. tamoxifen, C. thiazides.
- Testosterone increases the conversion of what to what? T4 to T3

Problem	Cause	Solution
Red Face	High estradiol	Decrease alcohol and/or caffeine, increase progesterone and/or zinc; avoid tight underwear and pants.
Acne	Increased sebum	Change diet: decrease milk, sweets, sugar and chocolate; decrease androgens
Hirsutism	Increased body follicle	Decrease DHT production
Feet edema	Increased salt retention	Increase potassium (1-3 gm QD) if there's no change, decrease androgens

Road Rage	Androgen overdose can cause brain edema which is an increase in GH deficiency	Decrease androgens and/or increase GH
Excessive libido	Too much testosterone changed to estradiol in brain; increase in androgen receptors in glans penis, scrotum and nipples.	Decrease androgens and decrease conversion of testosterone to Estradiol (E2)
Excessive erection	Too much DHT; increase in androgen receptors	Decrease dose of androgens and decrease conversion to DHT
Hair loss / Excessive body hair	Too much DHT	Finasteride 1 mg PO QD and eat less meat
Low Libido	Low estradiol	Increase testosterone and androgens
Impotence	Low DHT Elavated estradiol (E2)	Decrease estradiol (E2), increase testosterone and androgens
Peyronie's	Fibroid in penis; lack of DHT; possibly low cortisol	Apply DHT to penis, side of curve; if cortisol is low, small doses are ok; DHEA 20 mg-60 mg QD
Breast tenderness	Testosterone changed to E2	Give DHT and Anastrozole
Real gynecomastia	Testosterone changed to E2	Tamoxifen and decrease androgens
BPH	Testosterone changed to E2	Decrease caffeine and alcohol
Testicular atrophy	Elevated E2 (more often); elevated testosterone less often	Decrease E2 levels if no improvement, inject HCG 150 IU QD
Prostate Cancer/ Breast Cancer	Low testosterone and/or DHT	STOP testosterone. Take Q10 200 mg to 400 mg. If melatonin is low add melatonin. DHEA ok after PC, if DHEA does not react. Testosterone TX ok after 5 years.

Hormonal Intricacies #2

DHEA and Androstendiol

1. These are considered what type of hormones?
   a. Cross road hormones
2. Why?
   a. Because they will become other sex hormones
3. These have an effect on what body system?
   a. The immune system and connective tissue formation, i.e., ligaments and tendons.
4. Therefore, what is checked on the patient?
   a. If they have Lupus, MS, fibromyalgia, connective tissue disease, etc. (80% of pt.'s checked have low DHEA that have these diseases).
5. DHEA and Androstendiol are contraindicated in what condition?
   a. Sex organ cancers (they don't cause cancer, but will help the cancer grow).
6. Why?
   a. Because of their [DHEA and Androstendiol ability to convert into sex hormones and feed the cancer/tumor.
7. How can DHEA be increased naturally?
   a. Paleolithic diet
8. What nutrients decrease DHEA?
   a. Alcohol, caffeine, sweets, pasta and milk.
9. What hormones increase DHEA?
   a. Test, DHT and thyroid.
10. What hormones decrease DHEA?
    a. Cortisol and oral estrogens.
11. When should the dose of DHEA be increased?
    a. When the patient is under stressful conditions
12. When should the dose of DHEA be decreased?
    a. When the patient is in an un-stressful condition.
13. What are the symptoms of DHEA overdose?
    a. Oily skin, acne, increased body hair, therefore, decrease sugar intake.

NOTE: High sugar intake leads to high conversion of sugar to fat which leads to increased oil (sebum) production which leads to acne. **

    14. High DHEA can lower what hormone?

        a. Cortisol

    15. Which can precipitate what?

        a. Hypotension

    16. DHEA + Alcohol + Caffeine =?

        a. Estrogen—due to aromatase of testosterone.

    17. Foods high in fiber steal what from the GI tract?

        a. Steroids—fiber traps steroids that would normally be reabsorbed in the bowel.

Pregnenolone

    18. Low pregnenolone levels cause what?

        a. Poor memory, decreased color vision, decrease in awareness, low energy, increased joint pain, increase in dry skin, decreased libido, low mood, increased anxiety and decreased thinking.

    19. A decrease in sex hormones can lead to what?

        a. Low pregnenolone

    20. An overdose of pregnenolone may cause what?

        a. Nightmares and increase of sex hormone production

Aldosterone

    21. Low aldosterone levels cause patients to feel how?

        a. Like a "zombie"

    22. Patients feel better when?

        a. When lying down

    23. What do they experience when they are standing?

        a. Vision focus problems

    24. What other symptoms are evident?

        a. Salt cravings, polyuria, low blood pressure, hollow dehydrated look, teeth marks are left on tongue and skin "tenting".

    25. How is a low aldosterone level treated?

        a. Fludrocortisones 0.05 mg to 0.2 mg QD

    26. It is contraindicated in whom?

   a. Patients with easy leg edema
27. One can increase the aldosterone levels by doing what?
   a. Eating salt, drinking water and moving around—DON'T STAND OR SIT TOO LONG!!!

Prolactin, LH, FSH

28. Elevated prolactin levels indicate what?
   a. Deficiency in sex hormones and elevation of LH and FSH
29. LH is elevated when?
   a. During the 13/14th day(s) of the menstrual cycle
30. Low Sex Hormone Binding Globulin (SHBG) =?
   a. Low Estradiol (E2) or T3 deficiency or high androgens
31. High Hormone Binding Globulin (SHBG) =?
   a. High T3 or low androgens and/or GH
32. How can we "boost" sex hormones?
   a. An organic Paleolithic Diet
33. What should be avoided?
   a. Caffeine, soft drinks, pasta, whole grains, bread, bran and milk products.
34. What must be done?
   a. Lose weight (NO OBESITY)
35. Men must avoid what?
   a. Tight fitting underwear
36. All patients should avoid what?
   a. Chronic stress and smoking of any kind

Strong Stimulators of E2/P4	Strong Inhibitors of E2/P4
GH	
Cortisol at low doses	Too much Cortisol
Thyroid at low doses	Too much thyroid

Estrogen/Progesterone

37. Typical estrogen complaints and signs are what?
   a. Vaginal dryness, hot flashes and flabby breasts

38. What's the solution?
    a. Double the dose of Estradiol (E2) using the "1/2 method" (see previous notes).
39. A short menstrual cycle with droopy breasts is caused by?
    a. Low estrogen
40. A short menstrual cycle with swollen breasts is caused by?
    a. Low progesterone (P4)
41. A long menstrual cycle with droopy breasts is caused by?
    a. Low estrogen
42. Being depressive with low energy is caused by?
    a. Low estrogen and catecholamines
43. Being premenstrual depressed is caused by?
    a. Low estrogen and catecholamines and catechol estrogens.
44. Menstrual hot flashes are caused by?
    a. Low estrogen
45. Droopy breasts are caused by?
    a. Low estrogen
46. Small breasts are caused by?
    a. Low estrogen from childhood
47. An estrogen overdose may cause?
    a. Nervousness, tension, anxiety, outbursts of anger, painful menstruation migraines pre-menstrually and swollen painful breasts.
48. What's the solution?
    a. First: double the dose of progesterone (P4)
    b. Then: decrease the estrogen.
49. Heavy menstrual bleeding is caused by?
    a. An excess of Estradiol (E2) or a progesterone (P4) deficiency.
50. What's the solution?
    i. Give a dose of progesterone (P4) the first 14 days of the menstrual cycle then double the dose the last 14 days of the menstrual cycle, i.e., Days 5-14 give 100 mg and Days 15-28 give 200 mg.
51. Why?

    a. B/C progesterone is produced in the ovaries and naturally rises during the latter half of the menstrual cycle and we are wanting to mimic the menstrual cycle.

52. Uterine fibroids are caused by?
    a. Long term progesterone (P4) deficiency

53. Cysts in the breasts are caused by?
    a. Long term progesterone (P4) deficiency with elevated estrogen levels

54. Large breasts are caused by?
    a. Low progesterone (P4) deficiency with elevated estrogen levels

55. If a patient is taking progesterone and they are not receiving the progesterone effect, what's too high?
    a. Estrone (EI)

56. What's the solution to this?
    a. Give D:M
    b. Change from oral estrogen to topical estrogen

57. Progesterone does what?
    a. It will convert Estrone (EI) to Estradiol (E2), which cause a more estrogen effect.

58. If the patient is experiencing a "roller coaster" effect progesterone therapy, what should be done?
    a. Check the diet, i.e., decrease sweets intake, carbs and increase boiled/steamed meats and veggies, respectively, and avoid fruits for 2-4 days
    b. Check vitamin D

REMEMBER: If the patient uses skin lotion, it can block hormone absorption. ** ****REMEMBER: Three types of breast pain—a, sides of breast = too much P4; b. inside/center of breast = too much estrogen; c. sensitive nipple(s) = too much testosterone.

59. If a patient is suffering with menorrhagia, what should be done?
    a. Increase the progesterone during the latter of the menstrual cycle (days 14-28) double as needed

60. If a patient has cyclical migraines and droopy breasts, what is to be given?
    a. Estrogen and progesterone

61. If a patient has cyclical migraines and breast tenderness, what is to be given?
    a. Progesterone ONLY
62. Swollen breasts are caused by what?
    a. Low progesterone
63. Swollen, puffy face, swollen calves, hands and feet is caused by?
    a. Low thyroid
64. Swollen feet and ankles are caused by?
    a. A low protein diet
65. Muscle cramping is caused by?
    a. Low magnesium
66. Muscle weakness is caused by?
    a. Low potassium
67. Hypertension in the evening is caused by?
    a. Low cortisol

Testosterone in Women

Low Testosterone Signs and Symptoms	
Nervousness	Lack of Interest
Depression all day	Dry skin
Anxiety	Urinary incontinence
Fears	Low libido
Low stress tolerance	Low orgasm
Hysterical reactions	Low nipple sensitivity
Lack of mental firmness	Painful intercourse
Submissive	Lack of body hair
Hypochondrial	Pale
Abdominal obesity	Lack of sexual body scent
Hot flashes	Poor muscle tone
Fatigue	Thighs w/ cellulite
	Varicose veins

NOTE: For females—if all other hormones are in high normal range, give 6 mg of testosterone daily 3 mg in am and 3 mg in pm. Start with 2 mg per day (1 mg in am and pm) and increase by 1 mg daily every 60-90 days.

68. How is testosterone in women "boosted"?
    a. Paleolithic diet
    b. AVOID: alcohol, vinegar, caffeine, and sugar, soft drinks, cookies, and bread, pasta, cereal and milk products.

When to Lower Test Dose	When to Raise Test Dose
High protein diet	Low protein diet
High fat diet	High cereal diet
High calorie diet	Low calorie diet
Low physical activity	Diarrhea
	High physical activity
	High stress
	High thyroid function/levels
	Oral estrogens
Excessive Testosterone Signs	
Oily skin	Authoritative
Acne	Excessive muscle development
Oily hair	Male pattern baldness
Excessive sex drive	Excessive body hair
Excessive clitoral swelling	

69. Solution to acne?
    a. Decrease sweets intake
    b. Decrease androgens
70. Solution to feet edema?
    a. Increase potassium
    b. Decrease androgens
71. Solution to painful engorged clitoris and excessive libido?
    a. Decrease androgens
72. Solution to male pattern baldness and excessive body hair?
    a. Decrease testosterone dosages
    b. Eat less red meat.

NOTE: If the patient has side effects of swelling, oily hair, body hair overgrowth THINK: wrong food intake, i.e., high salt or obesity

**NOTE: It is important to know that too much of any androgen can first raise the other androgens, but, in the long run, will depress the other androgens.

Frequently Asked Questions

Question: What is the test? How do you do the test?

Answer: Knowing your saliva hormone levels is how we assess if your hormones may be out of balance and we use these test during treatment to determine if your current natural hormone regimen is working for you. If you are wondering whether certain symptoms may be due to a hormone imbalance, this is a quick, easy, and accurate way to find out. Basically you have to spit into a testing tube and fill it about half way up.

Question: What happens after the results come in?

Answer: We look at the questionnaire about your symptoms and then reference the lab results. I see that you've got this, this, this and this symptom. Well, this symptom correlates with this hormone and look, it's low. Or you have this other problem. We'll go back and forth letting you know exactly what is wrong. Then we'll tell you we're going to start you on a program—if you need it. Not everybody needs it.

Let's just say you're that person who needs progesterone—we're going to give you a syringe, that has cream inside. So what you do is you push it from this line to this line. This one is 100 mg of progesterone per ml.

For men, for example, we'll give you testosterone or DHEA or one of the other hormones that we talked about. You press the plunger and take out 1 cc-that's 100 mg. You apply it onto the skin, we recommend that you rotate the sites, inner arm, sides of body and inside of the thigh. So Monday, Tuesday, Wednesday, Thursday, Friday, Saturday, Sunday, you just keep going around the world. Usually after a warm shower or bath when the skin is supple because it allows for absorption. Let's take one symptom that correlates with a particular hormone—progesterone—insomnia. You put on the 1cc all of a sudden you come back to us and say you know, it's better but I want it better, the magic word is complain.

Complain. In about 3 or 4 days if you don't see a significant increase in your sleeping habits, complain. Because you'll call me and you'll say you know, I don't think this is working. I'll say what's happening? Well, I'm sleeping an hour more than I used to but I'm only sleeping 3 hours a night. You don't have enough progesterone. It was low you're not getting your level high enough so use 2 lines.

With you constantly talking to us we keep increasing your dose depending on what symptom you have. Then all of a sudden you've got to 3 lines and you say to us, you know I slept for 8 hours, I haven't slept for 8 hours in I don't know how long and the next morning when I woke up I was so tired, I felt like I didn't sleep at all. Cut it back. If 2 lines didn't do but 3 lines was too much, take 2-1/2 lines.

We have people that are so in tune with their symptoms that they know exactly how much of each hormone to adjust. Little by little they come back to us and they say, I want it all separate. I want the DHEA separate, I want the testosterone separate, I want to tweak it myself.

We say okay. So we separate everything then she says, I need 1 line of progesterone, I need a 1/2 of the line of estrogen, I need 1/4 of the line of testosterone and 2 lines of the DHEA. That's what makes me feel good. Okay. Can you mix it all together? This one adds up to this, this one adds up to that, i make up all the formula, put it all into one syringe. All you use is 1cc of this and you have everything that you wanted in there. Cuts down the cost. Those tubes for every cc is about $1 so if you need 60 of them twice a day that's $60.00 a month. If you need 2 prescriptions that would be $120.00. So what we want to do is cut it down. It might be a little on the expensive side in the beginning but if you complain and you help us, we can probably bring it down to one syringe that's got everything in it, 1cc a day that's all you need. We have a lot of patients, we've brought it down to about $40.00 a month. We have another patient that's about $100.00 a month because they want to really fine tune everything. But it's up to you. If you have insurance the insurance will pay and all you have to pay is your co-pay. You get two prescriptions the estrogen combo and the progesterone, you get 2 co-pays. Three prescriptions, you needed testosterone, for libido for example. We make testosterone cream for woman, for example, that have a problem orgasming, and it works. That's a separate prescription. What you want, you let us know.

Does this make sense? Don't you think that everything should be like this. I think all prescriptions should be like this so they can fine tune it to the patient.

Question: What if you have all the hormones at the right level?

Answer: You mean to tell me that all the hormones are at the right level and you have a ton of symptoms. I have yet to find that person. We've tested thousands of patients and we have yet to find that patient. Now we did find a patient that was going to the emergency every single month for Sjögren's disease. We studied her and it was not only the hormones but it was lack of vitamins. They were missing 14 different elements between vitamins and hormones. When we replaced them that lady went from going to the hospital emergency room once a month with heart inflammation to maybe once a year.

Question: Just had a baby a year ago and have asthma, will this help?

Answer: If you have asthma, progesterone is a muscle relaxer so it will allow the smooth muscles in the bronchioles to relax and allows for better breathing. Isn't it interesting we have some patients that come up to us and say, I didn't have asthma until I went into perimenopause and started having hormone problems? Had they had enough progesterone earlier in life and now the lack of it the cause of the asthma?

Question: Can I take the test if I'm on birth control pills?

Answer: If you're on birth control pills, you have to write that down. Birth control pills are like synthetic hormones. We'll ask you what brand you're on so we can consult our records.

Question: Can I take birth control pills and natural hormones together?

Answer" No. Get off the birth control pill, use alternatives and balance your hormones.

Take the test, let us know exactly what you're taking, just the name of the medication and we'll deduce exactly what's in there. So the first thing we do when a person is on synthetics is and if it's not for birth control, these are not for birth control pills, these hormones are for helping fertility. I'm just saying that these hormones will make you more fertile. We've had a lot of patients that we've actually helped get pregnant. Do the test, tell us what you're on, let us know how you're feeling, then we'll supplement her with a formula . . . if she's telling me I don't have any headaches, I don't have any breast tenderness, I really don't have any symptoms on this, we try to make the natural hormone as close in formula or strength to the synthetic she's taking. If she said to us I'm on the synthetic but I'm having headaches and I'm having breakthrough bleeding and I'm having bloating, then we know that we first have to figure out the formulas as is and then we put into consideration that even with this she still has break through bleeding, therefore we need to add more progesterone.

Profuse bleeding. The endometrial lining is not being held, that's not enough progesterone. We've had a lot of patients, I told you some of the easier stories. I had patients that were 21 years old which to us after they've had a full hysterectomy and the patient comes in and says I had a full hysterectomy. Why? I was bleeding 14 days out of the month. What happens is that's anovulatory cycle. What happens is the brain sends down a hormone (FSH) to the ovary . . . the messenger is called a follicle stimulating hormone, this is the same hormone that causes hot flashes. The follicle starts to mature and it starts to grow. By day 14 it starts to look like a grape and spikes a high amount of estrogen. The high amount of estrogen going to the brain sends another hormone back called luteinizing hormone. The luteinizing hormone causes that grape to break. If you ever bit into a grape and pulled out the seed, that little seed is what can get you pregnant. The resulting grape, as it starts to turn into a raisin, the liquid that's coming out of that grape, that's progesterone. So the progesterone rises and fall over the next 14 days. The people that don't have this spike in estrogen will never cause the release of luteinizing hormone therefore they won't make any progesterone. So there is no progesterone to maintain the uterus and she bleeds for 14 days. We supplement with estrogen to help this happen and then progesterone to help maintain the womb. Person goes from bleeding for 14 days for a couple of years to having a baby. They joke up in Carefree that Rudy's getting all these people pregnant. No . . . No . . . all I did was help with the hormones.

Question: Can I collect the saliva anytime?

Answer" It's got to be the first morning saliva. Plan a 1/2 hour of spitting. A little bit of lemon or something you've got to smell. But plan on just sitting there.

Question: What happens if I just can't make saliva?

Answer: If you can't do saliva, then go to a doctor and get a blood test but be careful.

When men go for a testosterone blood test, their going to check total testosterone. You must get the free testosterone. The total testosterone would be bound to the steroid hormone binding globulin and give a false reading.

Question: So what test should we ask for?

Answer Free testosterone. Total testosterone or Free testosterone and both. And Free.

Question: What happens if I have a running nose?

Answer: It won't. Because what will happen you will be able to tell one from the other. One when it comes to the back of the nose you'll swallow it. You'll be able to spit in the jar, don't worry about that. It's a real pain to do it but it is the most reliable way to get hormones because the only way you get hormones into the saliva is the spillage from the blood. The only way to spill from the blood is for it to be free unbound.

Question: Who do I talk to if I already have results of tests?

Answer: A doctor.

Question: Do you know a way to make sure we have enough saliva?

Answer It's a problem here in Arizona. Because everybody is so dry. That's why I say 3 days beforehand if you really hydrate yourself well, more salty foods, more water, a gallon a day will decrease your aldosterone hormone that keeps the water in your system. This will help you make saliva.

Question: Do I have to take hormones every day?

Answer: Progesterone. If your cycling on a regular basis you may need a little bit of progesterone for estrogen symptoms, that I don't want to get into in front of everybody right now, right off the bat you'll need progesterone, there's no doubt in my mind. What we need to do is find the right dose and once we find the right dose you may not even be supplemented for the whole month. You might take one cc for the first 14 days then double up to 2 or 3 cc for the last 14 days. We have some patients that will actually use the progesterone during their period. If you had a period and it was very achy, bloaty and irritating, and you applied a little of progesterone you'll slow down the bleeding. It will last a little longer instead of being 5 days, you'll be at 7 days but without heavy bleeding and without any pain.

Question: What was the name of the hormone that controls water?

Answer: Aldosterone. It's another hormone. It is what keeps the salt tension and the bodies blood pressure up.

Looking at the hormone pathways we find if I gave you this hormone, and gave you enough of it, not only would you raise your level of this one but it would be converted to other next to it, it will branch out. DHEA is one of those hormones. Progesterone is one of those hormones that will become other hormones if you saturate it Now I want to think of your body as a glass. Until you fill the glass, nothing will spill out. So if you're deficient in progesterone, once you fill the progesterone some of it may be converted to another hormone. But until you fill it, it won't. The same thing with the salvia. Sometimes people come back to us and say I took another saliva test and I got a result of 30,000. What we're measuring is what spills. So if you had this full cup and I drew a drop out, that's what we're measuring. If I took my whole hand full and wrung it out and I saw ten times what that drop was it would seem like an enormous amount. But compared to the whole cup of what's in your body it's not a lot. So even levels of 30,000 in the saliva don't scare us.

Question: Is it true that being cold all the time is a hormone imbalance. My doctor says I'm fine.

Answer: Low thyroid. There's nothing that's been proven about that. Now you understand what I'm talking about. So what you have to do is find a physician that also understands because what he'll do, we have some physicians you can talk to, what'll happen is, Dr. Carlos Santos or Dr. Lee, what he'll do is give you a certain amount of armour thyroid and we want you to keep measuring your temperature and let's say you on 1/2 a grain of armour thyroid and you take it for a month and all of a sudden from 94's you're up to 96. So he says okay let's go to one grain. You go to one grain and all of a sudden you're at 97.6 under the arm temperature. That's it, that's your dose. Understand that we're mostly water. To increase the body temperature by 1 degree on 100 kg person, like myself, burn. You have to burn 1,000 calories just to increase and keep that 1 degree more. So what happens to that food you eat? 1,000 calories gets burned. That's why most of us stay skinnier when we're younger.

Question: Can you have a regular cycle and be less than a month. I have a period every 15 days.

Answer: You could have a 21 day cycle, you could have a 25 day cycle it depends on the individual. 15 is a bit short. But usually what you do is you want to find where that peak of estrogen is, if a person has got a 25 day cycle, so back 14 days and that's where the peak is. So when you begin to bleed it's usually 14 days earlier was ovulation. So if your cycle shortens if s because of lack of progesterone.

Question: What do most doctors say about this.

Answer: I've had a couple of bouts with some endocrinologists as you could think. I'm a pharmacist and their doctors. They'll get on my case and I'll say what is the difference between any person as long as they sat there and they learned. Because I don't have a degree that says doctor, I didn't go through that route, but I spent the last several decades reading books and studying. I can do my own case study.

I'm going to talk to you now about something called a coffee enema. I don't know if you ever heard of it. If you take organic coffee and you brew it and you use it as a normal enema—4 to 6 cups for the normal adult—you bring it into your colon and you let it sit there for about 15 minutes then you release it what happens is, the Amish people, for example, use it to fight cancer. Until 30 years ago the coffee enema was in AMA's Merc index. Until they took it out they went the naturopathic way. What does it do, okay the naturopaths decided to study more about it Regular doctors say that it's like giving you a high dose of caffeine so it makes you feel better, it really doesn't do anything.

Naturopaths claim there are three things that it does, one—it cleans out the colon, gets rid of toxins that circulate into the liver. Anything you have in the intestinal tract gets absorbed into the blood. As it gets absorbed into the blood it first goes into the liver, the liver goes through a filtering process. All the impurities that it doesn't want gets put into the gall bladder then the intestine. Normally, it goes out in the stool. Normally. Sometimes, it can't clean it as well so it keeps circulating back and forth, back and forth, in and out, in and out, never actually getting rid of it. We call this entero hepatic circulation. The older you get, the less that your liver will work, the higher degree that that happens, the more allergies you get. The liver is dirty. Impurities get absorbed by the blood in the intestine, taken out by the liver, re-introduced into the intestine and re-absorbed.

Question: Can you explain how hormones and ratios of hormones play a part in rebuilding my body?

Answer: Sure, for arguments sake let's say perfect balance and levels of hormones was 100. So regardless of the hormone, all hormones need to have a level of 100. To simplify the matter even more, let's say you only have 4 hormones. DHT which when it exerts its influence causes baldness. Now we have a male or female that is complaining of hair loss. The other 3 hormones progesterone's, estrogen, testosterone are no longer at 100. They are less. Let's say 50 men or woman may figuratively be at 50,50,50 but if the DHT stays at 100, it will influence the scalp more and the patient will lose hair.

Question Some hormones can be bought over the counter and they are naturals. Why can't I just take those?

Answer Well for the first part OTC hormones are not regulated. They are considered a food and therefore can contain discrepancies from what is on the label and the true concentration. So even buying the same brand may vary in the amount you get from batch to batch. So regulating you could be a nightmare. Second Where's the testing to make sure your low. Several symptoms may be for hormonal deficiency as other diseases. Thirdly, we have the problem with hormonal steroid clearance. The body has threshold of the total amount of all hormones and when surpassed, the body (liver) will begin to indiscriminately begin to clear. Remember this is figurative.

To be able to visualize and simplify a much more intricate reaction we call metabolism of hormones. But we have to start somewhere. Let's define a new body that only has 4 hormones. Also, let's say that the hormone right level for each of the hormones is 1, 2, 3, 4. So that if we were to graph it, it would look that each hormone would be larger than the previous one. Almost like stairs. Now, in this particular body, we will add up all the levels 1+2+3+4=10. That's our hormonal load. Now let's say I go to the vitamin store and take hormoneX which normally should have a level of 4 and bring it up to 10 because I really don't know the dose to take. I don't even know the purity of the substance I'm taking.

What happens? Well the body will start to clear the hormones and as it does, it reduces across the board to bring the load back to 10. If you keep introducing that hormones and go beyond that level, other hormones will be destroyed. So again, figuratively speaking, if you were to increase to 10, the body would reduce all the hormones which would mean that the hormone who would have a level of 0. The hormone that was a level of 1 would be totally lost. The process of metabolism is much more complicated than this but it will allow you to visualize the introduction. A lot of one hormone can suppress the production of other hormones. In practice we can use this to our advantage to treat disease.

PCOS is a disease that cysts in the ovary. Cause high amounts of testosterone to be produced giving a woman many manly features. By giving her the right progesterone and estrogen in the normal ratio, but higher dose, you will decrease the testosterone over time, cause the body to be built in a more womanly fashion.

Hormonal tension—Let's say we poured 1 pound of salt and 5 inches. Then let's pour the same amount just closer together. Not so close that there is only one mound, but close enough that the two mounds touch. This would cause the both peaks to be higher. Let's say 7. So it is with hormones if you increase a particular hormone you will immediately increase the hormones it metabolized to and also increase the level that the particular hormone metabolizes from, because you will have to use less of the precursor hormone since the level of the hormone we're talking about is already high.

An interesting fact is that as we get older our hormones and vitamins all decrease, yet our cholesterol increases. I explain this as if the body was a car manufacturer. In the beginning we're making 1000 cars a day (hormones) and we need 4 tires for every car (cholesterol). So we have a standing order from the factory for 4000 tires every day. Now we only make 500 cars but the standing order for the tires was never reduced. So over time, the tires (cholesterol) back up and their level increase.

I started this book by thanking God. I would like to end it by thanking my wife "Laurie Dragone" who with our four girls Jessica, Melissa, Christina and Alexa who have been God's greatest gift to me.

www.ingramcontent.com/pod-product-compliance
Lightning Source LLC
Chambersburg PA
CBHW031235280526
45784CB00004B/1588